SPECIAL DELIVERY

The life of the celebrated British obstetrician

William Nixon

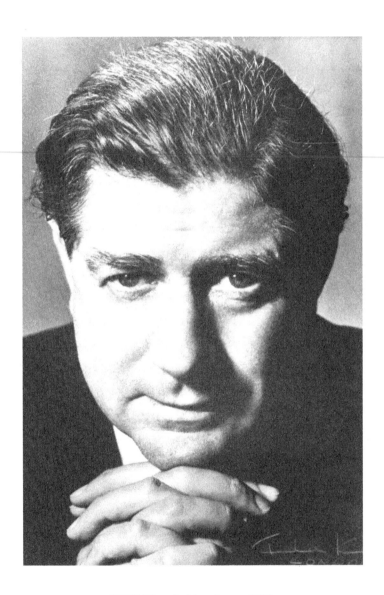

WCW Nixon in his prime at UCH

SPECIAL DELIVERY

The life of the celebrated British obstetrician

William Nixon

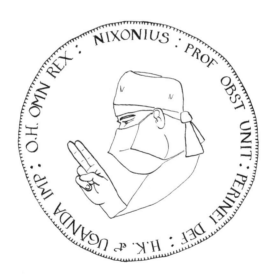

by

Geoffrey Chamberlain

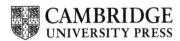

Shaftesbury Road, Cambridge CB2 8EA, United Kingdom

One Liberty Plaza, 20th Floor, New York, NY 10006, USA

477 Williamstown Road, Port Melbourne, VIC 3207, Australia

314–321, 3rd Floor, Plot 3, Splendor Forum, Jasola District Centre, New Delhi – 110025, India

103 Penang Road, #05–06/07, Visioncrest Commercial, Singapore 238467

Cambridge University Press is part of Cambridge University Press & Assessment, a department of the University of Cambridge.

We share the University's mission to contribute to society through the pursuit of education, learning and research at the highest international levels of excellence.

www.cambridge.org
Information on this title: www.cambridge.org/9781900364980

www.rcog.org.uk

Registered charity no. 213280

First published 2004

A catalogue record for this publication is available from the British Library

ISBN   978-1-900-36498-0   Paperback

RCOG Press Editor: Jane Moody

Design: Tony Crowley

CONTENTS

FOREWORD

Professor William Nixon directed the Obstetric Unit at University College Hospital (UCH), London, for twenty years from 1946 to 1966. These were innovative times in obstetrics and gynaecology and Nixon was among the innovators. Much that is now accepted as normal good practice was pioneered by him and today's management of pregnant women and their babies stems from his work. He was a humane doctor and he expected this of all who worked with him. Pregnancies come from two people and Will Nixon saw to it at UCH that both were recognised. Thoughtful treatment of father and mother were the norm. In both obstetrics and gynaecology, Nixon's researches led to new scientific ideas being introduced first at UCH, then nationally and in turn worldwide. Professor Nixon sent the men and women that he trained to all parts of the world and there they carried out his principles, which still live on.

I was a medical student at UCH fifty years ago. Falling under the Professor's influence I went into obstetrics and gynaecology for life. Now, in retirement from clinical medicine, I work in the History of Medicine Unit at the Clinical Medical School, University of Wales in Swansea, and have time to research and write about the life of my master.

Geoffrey Chamberlain,
Llanmadoc
Gower
2004

PREFACE

By SIR JOHN PEEL KCVO FRCP FRCS FRCOG
President of the Royal College of Obstetricians and Gynaecologists, 1966–1969

I first met Will Nixon when we were both applying for a consultant's post at the Soho Hospital. He got the job – rightly, because, although a year younger, I had started medicine much later than usual for a variety of reasons and so was young in experience. He remained loyal to Soho and in the 1940–41 Blitz on London he dealt with air-raid casualties there. From the middle 1930s until his appointment at University College Hospital (UCH) in 1946 he gave the impression of being unsettled and spent long spells abroad in Hong Kong, Turkey and other places. In 1946 he succeeded FJ Browne to the only full time Chair in Obstetrics and Gynaecology in a London undergraduate teaching hospital, apart from the all female one at the Royal Free.

The following pages in this biography record the full extent of the work carried on in his department – teaching, training, research directed towards improving the wellbeing of patients in all aspects of maternity and child welfare. Many members of his team went on to occupy leading positions in obstetrics and gynaecology in the UK and abroad. His close collaboration with outside bodies and individuals engaged in maternity and child welfare was of considerable importance. As a Member of Council of the Royal College of Obstetricians and Gynaecologists, he contributed significantly in all aspects of its work.

One of his important achievements was to establish a Childbirth Research Centre at UCH, designed to raise funds for research. This had hardly got off the ground before his death. This body continued for ten years at UCH before it moved across to the Royal College of Obstetricians and Gynaecologists, where it has been ever since raising money for research purposes throughout the UK and abroad. This really was his last baby.

In all his years, Nixon had lived life to the full: "I will drink life to the lees" as Tennyson had written of Ulysses. I had known him in London as a fellow traveller in our professional progression but only got to know and appreciate aspects of his character to be admired in the last ten years or so of his life. In every aspect of his thinking and practice he was indeed *avant garde* – a true pioneer who laid foundations for his successors to follow. Outside his professional life he was a delightful host and companion. He entertained at the Savage Club and at his favourite restaurant, the Copper Kettle in Wigmore Street.

Colleagues, students and patients alike mourned him freely when he died, but he left behind a memory cherished by all who knew him.

Sir John Peel
Salisbury
2003

INTRODUCTION

Will Nixon was born a hundred years ago and died, far too soon, when he was still only 62. Yet his influence lives on and the force of his radical mind can still be felt. It is therefore fitting that one of his former students, Geoffrey Chamberlain, should write this book. For Nixon was not just a forward-looking and brilliant doctor, he was a human being with rare gifts of sympathy and compassion; a reformer in areas where medicine still lagged painfully behind and a crusader whose campaigns were to change for the better the lives of thousands of women. His personality was so strong that he gives people who never met him the perception that they knew him well.

There is hardly a cause which affects the welfare of women in which he did not make his impassioned views felt. He was a scientist who spoke from the heart. His principal aim was to change the art of midwifery into the science of obstetrics. He was a humanist who understood that the mind, nature, and sexuality of each woman must be constantly related to her problems and symptoms. He was thus a great trailblazer in his advocacy of what we now call holistic medicine. He was a first-rate clinician and an early advocate of the doctrine that women should govern the destinies of their own bodies. He was one of the first to arrange for his students to have lessons in birth control. It was then, it is hard to remember now, a pioneering move that caused raised eyebrows. He was equally adamant about the right of a woman to terminate her pregnancy if that was the right thing for her and her child. He acted as an expert witness in a number of celebrated legal cases, notably the Leon Uris libel action, when his obligation to examine women who had been the victims of the appalling Mengele experiments in Auschwitz affected him deeply.

He was an inspiring team leader who never tired of teaching his juniors to consider the woman first and her disease second. He was the most companionable of men, with a gift for friendship that transcended every barrier of creed and culture. He had particular empathy with the Jews and this was to be deployed with notable effect during his wartime years in Istanbul, when he helped many Jewish people to escape from Nazi persecution overland to Palestine. He was a notable champion of the British Council in Turkey and helped it export what is best in British culture and in particular our medicine. It was also while he was there, working by day in the wards and operating theatre, that he found the time and energy to pursue another parallel life in the shadowy world of British intelligence. He was a devout patriot and at the same time a convinced socialist who was eventually to find his true intellectual home among Jo Grimond's liberals. He believed in meritocracy, had a fervent faith in education, hated the old boy network, and loathed the class system.

Yet he was no puritan. No-one enjoyed more than he the good life. He loved wine, in particular his favourite Chateauneuf du Pape, and he was a personal friend of the great gourmet and wine authority André Simon. Perhaps because his professional life was so exacting, he much enjoyed the slightly louche ambience of the Savage Club. Never a rich man, with only his professor's salary to live on, he lavished his hospitality on visitors to his country from every part of the world. He had a particular affinity with the East, and relished his years in Hong Kong. Yet he never let his grasp of the wide horizons obscure his scrupulous care for his family. He criss-crossed England in his battered old Anglia, visiting schools in person until he found one suitable for his daughter. He chose St Mary's Calne, whose headmistress had run a school with distinction under Japanese occupation. Women traditionally fall for their gynaecologists; in Nixon's case the condition reached epidemic proportions and his daughter Wendie remembers receiving presents sent by her father's grateful female patients from all over the world.

In an era when there were still no professional fundraisers, he went from long, exhausting days in the hospital to equally taxing nights persuading wealthy industrialists to provide the capital for causes close to his heart. The central question which obsessed him was: why do so many babies die? As he remarked in a report that shocked the nation, if we had 50 deaths a week from air crashes we would do something about it. Since we lost them in childbirth we did not. His battle against this grievous waste of life was unrelenting, and he showed his unique gifts as an innovator in it. He appointed women doctors when they were still frowned on in many hospitals; he was a pioneer in inviting fathers to be present at the birth if they so wished. He even advocated the metric system in medicine long before it happened. His last words to his fellow doctors when he felt the onset of his third and fatal coronary were totally in character. He apologised for leaving an important meeting. One colleague expressed the hope that they had not embarrassed him. No, he told them; on the contrary, he was only leaving in case he embarrassed them. He went back to his office and died. That was the sort of man Nixon was.

Godfrey Smith

ACKNOWLEDGEMENTS

Writing a biography of this nature, the author is heavily dependent upon many people who either knew Will Nixon or could help with sources of reference. I am deeply indebted to his daughter, Wendie McWatters, who gave freely of her time and went to much trouble pursuing sources, travelling out to Turkey to explore the Istanbul time of her father's life. She also provided most of the personal photographs of William Nixon, together with much personal correspondence and printed memorabilia. Nixon has only one grandchild in medicine, Dr Marcus Harbord, who was also helpful in background work. Mr Godfrey Smith, columnist on the Sunday Times, kindly wrote the introductory profile and read the script, while Mr Oscar Turnill also read the manuscript and improved it by his suggestions. My wife, Professor Jocelyn Chamberlain, has read various drafts and improved them each time. Despite this checking, any errors that remain are mine.

Others have assisted me in many ways. Some who were on the staff of University College Hospital (UCH) with Professor Nixon have willingly helped, particularly Professor Dennis Bonham (and Nancie his wife), Professor Alan Boura, Professor Neville Butler, Jack Dumoulin, Professor John Martin, Richard and Barbara Law, Hebert Reiss, Rudi Saunders, Tony Woolf, Professor Dennis Hawkins. Others who were from UCH were Professor Denys Fairweather, Nixon's successor, Dr Pamela Bacon, Professor Richard Beard, Professor Robert Boyd, Principal of St. George's Hospital Medical School, Professor the Reverend Peter Curzon, Mr Elliot Phillip, the medical historian, Mr Don Menzies, Professor Norman Morris and Mr Christopher Nordin.

Other doctors who allowed me to intrude upon their time were Sir John Peel, Past President of RCOG (who also kindly wrote a preface for the book), Dr Howard Baderman, lately consultant in charge of the Accident and Emergency Department, UCH, Mr. George Bonney, lately orthopaedic surgeon of St. Mary's Hospital, the late Dr Amnah Murad, gynaecological surgeon, formerly of Baghdad. Also very helpful have been Professor Charles Rodeck, the current Professor of Obstetrics and Gynaecology at UCH, Dr John Blair of St. Andrew's University, Mr Richard Kerr Wilson, Consultant Obstetrician at Cheltenham, Professor Ho Kei Ma,lately of Hong Kong, and Professor Aykut Kazancigil of Istanbul. Dr Susan Williams, historian to the National Birthday Trust, helped me with the sequelae to Nixon's 1958 Perinatal Death Survey.

Most helpful with her memories was Mrs Nancy Chapman, Will Nixon's penultimate secretary.

In Malta I was assisted in my research into Nixon's early days by the Hon. A de Bono, Mark Brincat, Professor of Obstetrics and Gynaecology at the Royal University of Malta, and his wife, Margaret Brincat, the Reverend John Dimmock, Minister of the Scottish Church, and Dr Salvator Mousu, Director of Educational Services, National Trust of Malta.

A book like this needs the support of a lot of work done by librarians and archivists, who allow one more easily to get at records hidden on the shelves of libraries, and I am grateful to them for their help. The librarians of University College Hospital, University College London, the Royal Society of Medicine, the Royal College of Obstetricians and Gynaecologists and of the Central Library in Swansea were helpful in this country, as well as those of the National Bibliotheca in Malta. Miss Patricia Want, lately librarian at the RCOG, helped with document identification at the National Archives. The archivists who gave their help were those of the RCOG, St. Mary's Hospital Medical School and Alan Scadding, archivist to Epsom College.

Much of the photographic material came, with permission, from WCW Nixon's papers and from his family. All were enhanced and reproduced by Howard Whitehead and Richard Waters at the Medical Illustration Department of Singleton Hospital, Swansea. I have endeavoured to find the copyright ownership of most material. If any has been missed, I apologise. Contact me and any omissions will be corrected in future printings of this book.

I am also grateful to the large number of men and women who knew William Nixon and were able to pass on material. My thanks are to my forgiving secretary, Mrs Caron McColl, who decoded my handwriting and provided the many drafts so expertly. The publishing house of the College, particularly its head, Jane Moody, have worked hard to produce this volume, and to them I am grateful for their support and effectiveness.

Geoffrey Chamberlain

CHAPTER ONE

Early Days (1903–1918)

"You waves, though you dance by my feet like children at play,
Though you blow and you glance, though you purr and you dart;
In the Junes that were warmer than these are, the waves were more gay
When I was a boy with never a crack in my heart"

The Meditation of an Old Fisherman (1886)
WB Yeats

Malta was a comfortable island for British expatriates to reside in the 1900s. Britain had ruled for a century since helping to expel the French. Having been the shuttlecock of warring nations for long before that, Malta became an important dockyard facility for the Royal Navy, first for its sailing ships and later as a coaling station. Trade flourished during the Crimean War and particularly benefited from the opening of the Suez Canal twenty years later. The long sea routes round Africa were cut so that communications between Britain, India and Australia were reduced by many days. The island offered one of the best natural harbours in the Mediterranean and the Royal Navy soon appreciated this. Five dry docks were opened there. The Royal Navy was the largest industry on the island, with up to a third of the population employed either directly or indirectly by the British Armed Services. Any British civilians, such as the Nixons, lived in the reflected glory of this.

At dawn on Sunday, 22nd November 1903, after a long night, William Nixon was born at his parents' home at 22 Strada Leone in Floriana in Malta.[1] At this time his father, William Nixon senior, was 34 and his mother, Melita, was 22 years old. He had gone out to Malta from Nottinghamshire and she was born there.

William Nixon senior came from a long line of yeoman farmers who had been landowners in South Nottinghamshire for three centuries. There are fourteen William Nixons buried in turn in the old churchyard at Bradmore. William Nixon senior, born in 1869, was the eldest of six children; his father disappeared to America and William Nixon had to get a job and stand on his own feet. He became an apprentice engineer. At the time of William Nixon Junior's birth, he was a lecturer in applied mechanics and mathematics at the

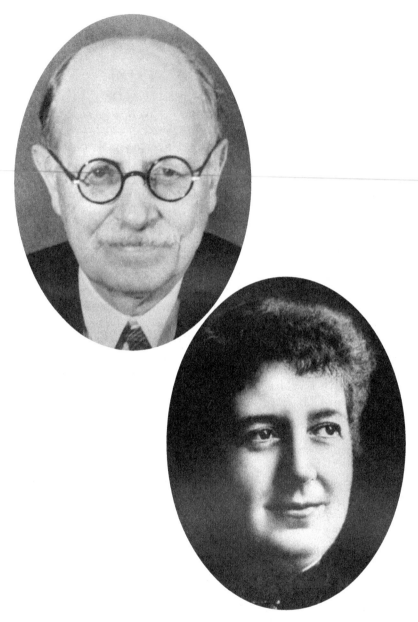

William Nixon Senior. Father of WCW Nixon and Melita Nixon, his mother;
taken about the time that WCW Nixon went to England to Epsom College (1915)

Apprentice College in the Naval Dockyard. Lord Strickland, the Governor of Malta, had conceived the idea of this Training Institute as a prestige engineering centre and insisted on an English teacher of mathematics. He brought Nixon out and appointed him (at £240 per year) to this position, from which he went on eventually to become the Principal.[2,3]

A major function of this College was the maintenance of the ten locomotives and thirty-odd carriages of the Malta railway, a six-mile long, narrow-gauge track going from Valetta to the Military lines at Imtarfa. Nixon senior took the railway to his heart and played a large part in its running, fighting against its eventual demise in 1934. The College at that time also trained men for the maintenance of the dry docks and other mechanics of the dockland. Nixon was appointed to the Royal University of Malta as Professor of Mathematics and then Dean of the Faculty of Engineering and Architecture – a combination of disciplines unique to this University.[4] He served that institution well for many years, returning to Britain before the Second World War.

Melita's father, Carl Riechelmann, had gone to Malta from Germany for political reasons. The family was very unhappy with the unification of Germany under Bismarck. He taught music and was the organist of the Presbyterian Church in Malta. Carl was also an active Freemason and was later a Grandmaster of the Lodge in Malta. He met, wooed and married Melita's mother, Marie Crowe, when she had gone to Malta on holiday. She had been a very good mezzo-soprano and was planning to become a professional opera singer but she gave this up on her marriage. With her husband, she opened an English High School in Valetta, of which no trace now remains. They returned to live in Maida Vale, London, for a few years but health reasons forced Carl and Marie Riechelmann back to Malta where the school was reopened. They had seven children, of whom Melita was the sixth.[4]

Melita and William Nixon senior had two children – William and Molly. William's life we shall trace in this book. Molly, who was also born in Malta, later came to London and studied mathematics at Bedford College.[5] There, Molly married a naval officer, Bradwell Turner, who achieved fame in World War Two when he, as a Lieutenant Commander, took HMS Cossack alongside and boarded SS Altmark, a Nazi prison ship, with cries of "The Navy's Here!" so rescuing the captains of the ships sunk by the Graf Spee in the South Atlantic, who were being held prisoner. He later rose to staff rank in the Royal Navy.

The house in Floriana where William Nixon was born still exists. It is a fine three-storied residence on the corner of Strada Leone and Britannia Street,

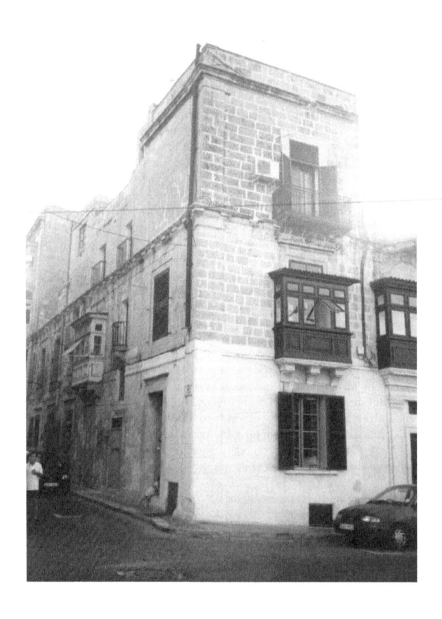

22 Strada Leone in Floriana, Malta where WCW Nixon was born and lived for his childhood years (Taken by Author 2002)

looking on to Independence Area, a large parade ground, which was previously used by the Armed Forces but is now a grassed football pitch. Floriana is at the base of the peninsula that contains Valetta, between Grand Harbour and Marsamxett Harbour, and was originally constructed as the outer landward defence of the capital of Malta. At the beginning of the twentieth century, Floriana was a suburb particularly favoured by British civilians who worked for the Maltese Civil Authority. The other end of the short Strada Leone comes out by the side gate of the Antonii Gardens, a cool walking place with fountains and the finest collection of ferns in the Mediterranean. At the time of Nixon's birth, this was the University Herbarium containing many descendants of the herbs used medicinally by the Knights of Malta three centuries before. Here, the child William must have played for many hours in his childhood. The booking office of the underground Floriana Station of the Malta Railway was on the edge of these gardens. Since Nixon senior was so closely associated with that railway, the family probably used this station frequently to go on trips inland up to Imtarfa. In Floriana, there were other botanical gardens, such as the Maglio, used by the Knights of Malta in the seventeenth century.

A few months before William Nixon's birth in 1903, King Edward VII had made an official visit to Malta. The Grand Fleet occupied the Grand Harbour in full strength, dressed overall, and the Royal Yacht sailed in with an impressive parade of barges and cutters to a background of gun salutes. He was entertained mostly by the Services, for there was a certain aloofness of the British towards the Maltese, keeping their own company and not mixing with the inhabitants of the Island. An official British Government report by General JJ Simmons, published a few years before William Nixon's birth, stated: "There was an almost absolute estrangement in society of the purely British from the native elements. This is very much regretted but is exceedingly marked; Maltese officers and gentlemen are not admitted to English clubs. There is also a strong anti-British feeling being engendered in secret, almost unknown to the British community".[6]

The British response to this report was muted; one reaction was the reformation of the Malta Fencibles, a section of the garrison made up of only Maltese soldiers. However, the divide between the Royal Navy and the natural citizens of Malta, based on snobbery, persisted until after the Second World War.

This was the slightly artificial atmosphere into which William Nixon was born and brought up as a young child. Nixon probably attended his grandparents' school for his first years but no records exist. The Upper Barrakka Gardens

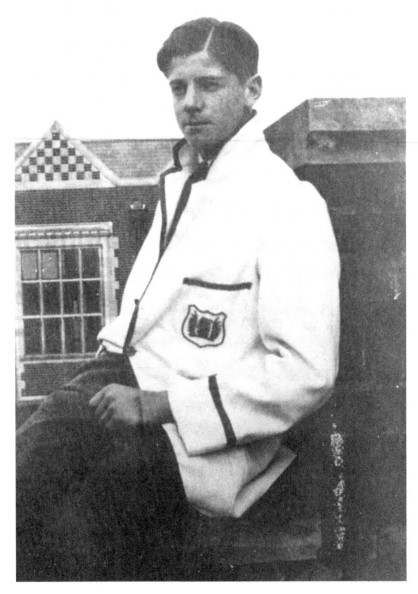

WCW Nixon at Epsom College. He was awarded his athletic colours which entitled him to wear the athletics blazer (1917)

were a short walk from his home. From here, the boy Nixon had a great view across the Grand Harbour. During the 1914–18 war, Malta was spared attack (unlike in the last War) and the harbour had a constantly changing scene of heavy battleships and light craft, particularly during the Gallipoli campaign of 1915. This would have enthralled young William, who was eleven when the war started.

In 1918, when Nixon was fifteen years old he was sent to England to finish his education. In 1920, his mother, fearing anti-German feelings, had William Carl Wallace, Nixon's name, changed by deed poll to William Charles Wallace Nixon. His schoolmates probably did not notice. He attended Epsom College and entered Carr House, where he became in turn a House and then a College prefect. He won his first XV school colours for rugby football, playing on the wing, and was a most popular member of the school. Nixon also boxed and played fives for the school, becoming Captain of Fives; during his tenure his house won the Fives Cup. He was also awarded colours in athletics, which entitled him to the honour of wearing an athletics blazer. He was made Head of House in his last year and in the Officer Training Corps he achieved top awards, being promoted to Sergeant.[7]

Nixon's academic record in school did not mirror his sporting activities. In his first year he was 16th out of 26. The following two years he was respectively 22nd out of 22 and 18th out of 19. In his last year he came seventh out of 17.[7] Either Nixon was a late developer or else schools in those days assessed their pupils on matters that were not important in later life; maybe schools still do.

Epsom College had strong connections with the London medical schools. William Nixon, after an interview with the Dean, Dr Charles Wilson, obtained a scholarship to St. Mary's Hospital Medical School, Paddington, in 1922 having passed his first MB examination at Epsom. Later in life, Alec Bourne, the noted gynaecologist at St. Mary's Hospital, claimed he had influenced Nixon. He knew him as a boy and when Nixon decided to go into medicine, pressed him to come to that medical school.[8]

CHAPTER TWO

The Medical Student (1922–1927)

Though you are in your shining days,
Voices among the crowd
And new friends busy with your praise,
Be not unkind or proud.

The Lover Pleads with his Friend
for Old Friends (1897)
WB Yeats

When William Nixon entered St. Mary's Hospital Medical School, it had been open for about seventy years. The hospital was part of the second wave of London teaching hospitals, the first being in the mid-seventeenth century. It is interesting that the new schools seemed to cluster along the axis of the Marylebone Road and many were associated with the London terminals of the major railway companies of that time (St. Mary's Hospital with Paddington, Middlesex Hospital with St. Marylebone, University College Hospital with Euston and the Royal Free Hospital with Kings Cross) so draining from the London Home Counties a wide hinterland of patients who could travel up to the outpatient departments. There were at this time twelve undergraduate schools in the capital and they all followed the same style of curriculum. All medical schools but one were traditional and heavily male-orientated in their selection of students, although some allowed a minority of women. They were also usually biased towards taking students from middle-class medical families. The exception was the Royal Free Medical School – then an all-women institution. The other schools thought at that time that male graduates would make the more reliable doctors and such blinkered selection was not eroded until after the Second World War.

The teaching of medicine has always been contentious and in the 1920s the debate was hotting up. The Government, the General Medical Council, the medical profession and the public were wanting their doctor to be a bit of a scientist but also to be a humanist; to be an all-rounder with some knowledge of everything that could go wrong with the human body and the ability to treat most of those problems. This produced a large number of general practitioners with a smaller layer of hospital-based specialists. Hence, medical training was aimed at this devil's brew.

London teaching hospitals were the ones that led in these traditions. Outside London, there were by now many provincial medical schools, which were in several aspects more progressive, but London stayed the traditional centre for producing good, well-rounded, middle-class male doctors. Each school had its own propensities: University College Hospital was renowned for its scientific training and those chosen to go there tended to be of a more intellectual bent. St. Thomas' Hospital took the social cream and St. George's Hospital was "… but a step down from the Club" at the bottom of Piccadilly. St. Mary's Hospital Medical School (SMHMS) put great emphasis on physical activity and particularly rugby football. It was said that the medical school, being just lateral to Paddington Station, the terminus of the Great Western Railway from Wales, made it easy for all the Welsh rugby players wishing to study medicine to pour off the train at Platform 3 and get into St Mary's. Rugby men from South Africa and Australia who wanted to be doctors also came to St. Mary's.

There had been no female medical students – indeed, except for secretaries and cleaners, women were not admitted to the student areas – but with the First World War, male doctors were being recruited into armed services and so St Mary's admitted the first female students in 1916. In 1924, while Nixon was a student, the Medical Committee of the Medical School decided not to accept any more women's applications. They felt that one of the reasons that the number of male applications was falling was because they preferred to go to medical schools where women were not taken.[1] St Mary's only took its share of female students in 1947 after the Second World War, when all London medical schools reassessed their gender discrimination (and the Royal Free Hospital Medical School admitted men).

St. Mary's Hospital Medical School in Nixon's time was in an inconspicuous building "hidden away in the space between the Hospital, the Great Western Terminus and the canal. It was as difficult to find as Meckel's ganglion."[1] There was a library as well as a student clubroom and restaurant in the basement of the New Wing. Some 300 beds in the hospital were available for student teaching and these were augmented by 700 at the affiliated hospitals in the region available for clinical teaching. The Princess Louise and Paddington Green Hospitals were brought into this group. Some students went to St. Mary Abbott's but the annexing of the Samaritan Hospital in Marylebone Road did not happen until after Nixon's student days. The advertisement in the contemporary Medical Directory boasted: "The hospital is in an extensive residential district in which students live and so avoid a daily wearisome journey to and from their work. A register of approved lodgings and private residences is kept for student accommodation".[2]

Student social life was restricted, usually by lack of personal funds, so entertainment was self-generated. The Music Society flourished, with a strong bias towards the operettas of Gilbert and Sullivan, performed in the library. Professional artists, mostly grateful private patients of the consultant staff, gave concerts. The Dramatic Society provided the medical students with an opportunity to get to mix with nurses openly and was enthusiastically supported in consequence. The Medical Society provided the site for distinguished visitors to debate. Arthur Conan Doyle on spiritualism and George Bernard Shaw on the Pathology of the Medical Profession were two such in Nixon's time.

Students arrived at a medical school bright-eyed and waiting to get their stethoscopes on someone's chest. They had visions of medicine conned from the books of Somerset Maugham and other predecessors of AJ Cronin and plays such as those of Frederick Treves. A slightly holy look would have been in Nixon's eye when he was accepted by St Mary's but then he found that the first two of the five years was to be spent on basic science, mostly anatomy, physiology and biochemistry. This was a damper and many medical students revolted against this. However, the professors of these preclinical disciplines held sway and their departments were powerful ivory towers, often completely divorced from the actual end product of making working doctors. Students learned detailed anatomy, for eighteen months dissecting cadavers, men and women whose bodies remained unclaimed by relatives when they died in the poor houses or mental hospitals. The curator who ran the dissecting rooms was a wizened man called Victor. He ruled that part of the empire, trying to contain the more extreme examples of gallows humour that medical students have. Nixon had to learn the minutiae of the body's muscles, its nervous system, blood supply and bony structures and many details besides.

Physiology was a little better; at least it dealt with function, which most students recognised as being more interesting than structure, but the whole syllabus was university-based with lectures (attended by up to fifty not very attentive students) and laboratory work, much of which was unnecessary for training as a doctor. Interest was often more focused on the bets made about the exact time that ash would fall from the cigarette permanently between the lips of a well-known lecturer, than the physiological content of the teaching.[3] There were no tutorials or seminars, now recognised as better ways of handing on information. Biochemistry followed suit and over the 1920s some new subjects were introduced into the curriculum. Epidemiology and medical statistics were yet to come; humanitarian subjects like sociology and psychology were shunned because they were not 'proper medicine'.

The Professor of Anatomy was John Frazer, a tall, commanding man who was a fine teacher. His book *Anatomy of the Human Skeleton* was the best British book on osteology and is still used today. Nixon obviously got on well with him for the professor invited him back to be a demonstrator when he was a candidate for the Primary Fellowship of the Royal College of Surgeons, a hurdle that could be taken in those days straight after second MB in the second year. Nixon impressed Fraser with his powers of understanding and the use of facts and principles. James Collingwood was the newly appointed Professor of Physiology. He had served in both the Boer and First World Wars and was very popular with the students as a precise, clear and logical teacher.

At St Mary's, Nixon would have to have been influenced by the new subject of immunology, as the chairman of that department was that giant of medicine, Almroth Wright, who developed and exploited therapeutic immunisation by vaccines. His work may not have attracted the students greatly but it was extensively used by the Government in the First World War when he introduced anti-typhoid vaccination into the army, with great success. Wright struck up a friendship with Bernard Shaw, who wrote *The Doctor's Dilemma* based upon Almroth Wright's discoveries and indeed portrayed him in the play itself. Wright expressed himself forcibly on roles for women in *The Unexpurgated Case Against Women Suffrage*, and in a notable clash at the Medical Society, Wright opposed Bernard Shaw in a debate favouring votes for women. The result of this debate between Man and Superman is not remembered but it was made famous by Shaw's remark, "He [AW] spoke such beautiful English it was not immediately apparent to everyone what rubbish he was talking".[4]

Alexander Fleming was in the Bacteriology Department. He was not a very strong teacher but full of kindness and of serendipity, having observed the effect that a penicillium spore, floating in by chance, had against pathogenic bacteria growing on blood agar in a Petri dish. This led to the production later of the first antibiotic, penicillin. Some detractors would say that this was luck, but luck only favours the prepared mind that can see the significance of such findings. In 1922, when Nixon joined the School, Fleming had discovered lysozymes, the natural antibiotic present in body fluids such as tears, and isolated penicillin in 1928. A Nobel Prize was awarded to Fleming after the practical use of antibiotics in World War II. These were the qualities of teachers in preclinical medicine who influenced Nixon.

Swimming and playing rugby football on the Athletic Ground in North Wembley leavened the preclinical years. The rugby players changed in a nearby pub at first but later in a temporary pavilion. After Nixon's time, St. Mary's Hospital had as many as five members of the England international rugby team playing in their hospital squad and they were invincible. In the 1920s, Medical School rugby was at a low ebb following the Great War and the team did not do well in the inter-hospital rugby cup. When Will Nixon joined the Medical School he had already played good rugby at Epsom and, having achieved a small reputation, he was put into one of the Medical School teams from his first year. He played in the pack as a lock in the scrum for most of his career, participating in some of the Hospital Cup matches but never on the winning side in the final of this knockout competition.

The St Mary's Hospital Medical School Gazettes of that time contain full accounts of the rugby team's games.[5] Criticism was freely given, with advice from the touchline from armchair journalists penetrating all areas. When Will Nixon was playing, the team contained two international players: Cussen, the

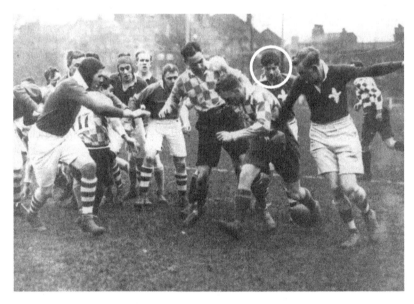

WCW Nixon (circled) playing for the St. Mary's XV. The scrum is just breaking up and a wing forward is trying to stop the opposition getting away with the ball. Nixon, lock forward is following up (1923)

Irish wing, and DN Rocyn-Jones, who played fullback for Wales and later was elected to the game's highest honour in Wales, President of the Welsh Rugby Union. The problem for other high-class student players was that London had several first class clubs, such as the Harlequins, Richmond and the London Welsh. Here, good players were welcomed and they could sharpen their skills against equally good opponents. Further, the selectors of national teams used to go to these games and would be more likely to spot good players in such matches. The temptation of divided loyalties was strong and several opted not to play for the Medical School in favour of hopes of a greater rugby career from being seen in these outside teams.

The Gazette's accounts of hospital rugby from 1922 to 1926 contain many references to Nixon, mostly complimentary, such as the occasion in March 1923 when, playing against the Harlequins XV, a certain try was prevented by his rushing back and touching the ball down in the face of heavy opposition. The price was a damaged elbow and Nixon had to leave the field. On another occasion that year, "Nixon showed what foot work could accomplish" and the following year Will scored under the posts after a long run – quite a feat for a big forward. Later, the forwards were complimented as being keen to work together, "… Nixon keenest perhaps of all".

Typical of the team's results while Nixon was playing was the season of 1924–25: played 25; won 15; lost 10; points scored 339; points against 159. This is a record of an active and successful side with an average of thirteen points for and six against in twenty-five games. In that year, games started to be played on Wednesday as well as Saturday afternoons.

As an all round athlete, Will was fond of most sports. He excelled at swimming and represented the medical school in swimming galas and also played for his medical school in water polo, a hearty game for those with robust physiques. He used to join the inevitable drink-together after the rugby game but was not very well off financially and did not stay. He used to describe how, for a treat of an evening, he and some mates would go to Paddington Station and share a long drawn-out cup of coffee.[6]

Having satisfied the examiners in the second MB examination, William Nixon moved on to the clinical aspects of his subject. The whole of clinical medicine was an apprentice art and students learned by watching doctors at work in the wards, outpatient departments and operating theatres. If one had a good teacher, one learned well. If there was a poor teacher, the result was less helpful. The hierarchy of consultancy was self-perpetuating. Established consultants commonly chose others to succeed them who had mirror-image personalities. In these circumstances, Nixon was greeted with a plethora of fine teachers, men who strode the heights of their subjects and were masters of not just the technical aspects of medicine but of all they surveyed socially. They left their stamp on St. Mary's Hospital students of Nixon's generation.

CA Pannett, one of the most able men at St Mary's Hospital Medical School, was the new Professor of Surgery. Other surgical teachers Nixon met were Warren Low, a well-liked surgical teacher who worked hard despite the disability of arthritis, which had started in the Boer War. Zachary Cope had returned from World War I, which he spent in Baghdad, in 1919 and was promoted to the full staff at St Mary's Hospital. He was a popular teacher and made some parts of diagnostic surgery easier with his little book, *The Acute Abdomen in Rhyme*. Cope was a short man and always had a wooden stool to stand on for operating (Mr. Cope's Box). He was quiet and calm in all things, a characteristic that made him unique among his surgical colleagues. Maynard Smith was a dapper man with a neat surgical technique, well remembered by students. Professor FS Longmead had recently been appointed head of the

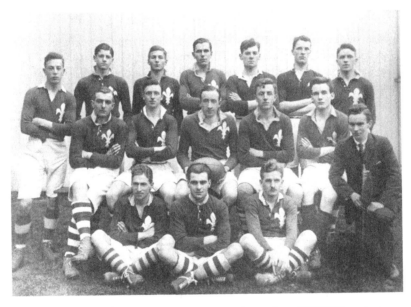

The St. Mary's Hospital Medical School Hospital Cup Team. WCW Nixon is second from the left in the back row. They did not win the cup (1924)

Medical Unit and had a high reputation among students. Other physicians who taught Nixon were Sir John Broadbent (a cardiologist) and Sir William Willcox, a kindly man who always took the underdog's side and hence was popular with students. The Dean, Charles Wilson, later Lord Moran, who went on to play an important part in maintaining Winston Churchill's health in the Second World War , was also an active teacher. As Dean, he personally interviewed and individually chose most of the students coming to St Mary's, including Nixon, over twenty-five years. Wilson considered that his personal choice of students was better than using the results of competitive examination or interviews by groups of senior doctors. Judging by the calibre of men coming out of St. Mary's Hospital in those years, he was right. Wilson usually interviewed by appointment in his Harley Street rooms and, while clearly interested in rugby-playing ability, he considered all good points of the men and a few women and chose discriminately.

The clinical training was basically six months each of surgery, medicine, obstetrics and gynaecology and twelve months of what were then called special subjects, which included a couple of weeks each in a basket of disciplines such as otolaryngology, paediatrics, dermatology, anaesthetics, psychiatry and the casualty department; pathology was slipped in amongst these clinical subjects. For the last six months, students devilled for individual house surgeons and physicians as they extended their apprenticeship. On the medical wards, the students were known as clerks while on the surgical wards they were dressers: both these terms being historic legacies from what medical students actually used to do in the century before; these now were but nominal labels. The students were divided into teams (firms) of three or four, each attached to an individual consultant. They were allocated a small number of patients by the registrar on the firm and were expected to see them daily, recording changes in progress and especially to attend ward rounds, which the chief usually did once a week.

Consultants usually arrived at the hospital in their fine cars at 1.45 p.m., having spent the morning at their consulting rooms in Harley Street, and were met at the front door by the team. At these ward rounds the consultant, with his attendant assistants, registrars, house officers and occasionally distinguished visitors, would move from bed to bed around the ward. At each bed a student would present the patient's history, clinical findings, treatment and progress. He was expected to remember every detail about his patients and would be quizzed about possible diagnoses and managements. This was often a shaking experience which frightened some students, as the consultants could be very aggressive and indeed, a few may even have taken pleasure in

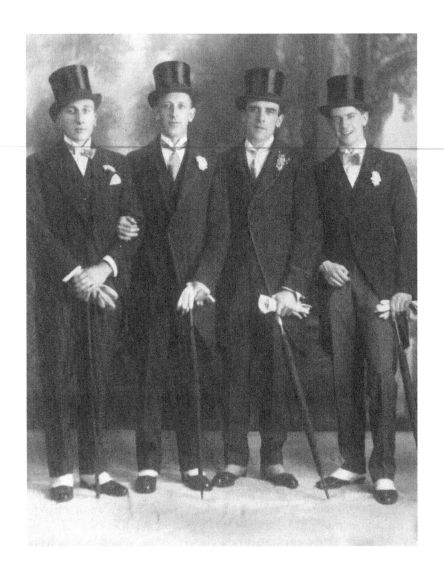

St. Mary's Christmas pantomime in 1927. Four budding surgeons. The students are JE Simpson, DM Murray, Charles Donald and WCW Nixon (on right)

humiliating young men. This minority of seniors seemed to be more intent on exercising the sharp edge of their tongues rather than in helpful teaching. The whole atmosphere of the St. Mary's Hospital Medical School at this time seemed to be determinedly non-intellectual or even anti-intellectual. The influx of students to the clinical years from Oxford and Cambridge (where only preclinical medicine was taught in those days) provided a much needed stimulation of talent. Some consultants seemed to think that mugging up the facts to get students through the examinations was enough.[3]

The comfort, and indeed the capacity to learn, on the wards of the hospital depended very much on the relationship each student made with the nursing sisters and their senior staff nurses. These women ruled the roost and if a student displeased them in the early part of their stay, the rest of their time on the ward could be very negative. It is almost certain that William Nixon, with his fine open face and his pleasant manner, steered his way skilfully through these shallows. One of the ways of earning grace was to be helpful on the wards. When the student left a patient, he made sure the bed was tidy and properly made to Sister's geometrical specifications, a quincunx of the sheets at the bottom corners of the bed. After the student had taken any samples, he returned the equipment to the right place and washed up all apparatus.

It was the task of one student, in rotation, to arrive on the wards half-an-hour early to sharpen the needles, which in those days were not disposable. This was done using a wine-bottle cork through which the needle was inserted obliquely so that ,when it came out at the bottom, the bevel was flat for the grindstone. This quite pleasant task was often accompanied by social chitchat with the more junior nurses and many a happy liaison started in this fashion in the mornings. The house surgeons, who had only just qualified, used to leave chits for blood to be taken and to be sent to the laboratories for tests. These blood samples had to be taken by each student from his own patients. This was a little traumatic at first; getting a needle into a vein is not always easy but practice made a little more perfect and by the end of the three years most medical students could take blood without too much bruising and pain.

The other major form of investigation with which Will Nixon would have dealt in the 1920s was X-rays. These had been introduced at the beginning of the century and had blossomed in the First World War; by the 1920s, diagnostic radiographs were an expanding new subject. They showed, with various degrees of clarity, gases, soft tissue and bone. The films had to be available in correct chronological order for the consultant's weekly round. Urine samples had to be checked, usually for protein and sugar, while some physicians used to insist upon inspection of the stools as a diagnostic measure of the functioning of the alimentary tract. This meant that the student had to ensure that, on the day the consultant went round, the sluice room contained a series of bedpans containing a recent sample stool of each of the patients he was looking after. Sometimes this involved very enthusiastic vocal encouragement in the wards for the hour or so before the rounds and caused much merriment among the other patients who were separated from the victim merely by thin cotton screens. All these practices of student life were still in place when the author studied clinical medicine at UCH twenty-five years later.

After general medicine and surgery, William Nixon studied six months of obstetrics and gynaecology. More emphasis was placed upon these subjects in Will Nixon's student days than it is now, for many students would become general practitioners and would be expected to deliver babies in the homes of their patients. In Britain then, only about one-fifth of women had babies in hospital under the care of consultant obstetricians, most of the rest delivering at home with midwives and the occasional supervision of the general practitioner. In the St Mary's Hospital Medical School district, however, home births had been diminishing since the end the War. In the 1920s, only about 400 births a year occurred at home, with 600 women delivered in hospital. A few women went to private nursing homes to give birth.

The senior consultant obstetrician in Nixon's student days was Thomas Stevens, who held a high opinion of Nixon's work and thought that he had acquired an excellent knowledge of midwifery and gynaecology. Stevens was a short man with a moustache and a neatly trimmed imperial beard who was a skilful surgeon and dogmatic teacher. The other obstetrician was Alec Bourne, who had spotted Nixon's talents already and encouraged his future ambitions. Both Thomas and Bourne considered Nixon to be a most agreeable student because of his personality and Bourne admitted later he was already grooming Nixon in the hope that he would join him as a consultant on the staff of St Mary's.[7]

If they were lucky, much of the real obstetrics was taught to the medical students by midwives, who were good at dealing with the normal and spotting the abnormal when it occurred. Alec Bourne was unhappy with this chance method of instruction and arranged for some students to go for two weeks to Queen Charlotte's Maternity Hospital. There, they were actively taught the art of obstetrics in the labour rooms by the resident medical officers (senior house surgeons). Some also went to other referral hospitals, the acme being the Rotunda Hospital in Dublin.

This subject, with its emotional aspects, was one where the student assumed some responsibility for what transpired, and it fascinated Nixon. He was always prepared to listen to and talk with people, showing sympathetic feelings and giving words of comfort. His ambitions to become an obstetrician began then. Probably it was his natural sense of humanity in seeing the women of Paddington in labour that turned his mind towards obstetrics. He decided then and stayed steadfast to this subject for the next forty years.

Gynaecology in the 1920s was mostly a surgical subject. Hormone treatments had not started and antibiotics to check infection were thirty years away; operative correction of problems was the norm. The practical teaching of gynaecology to mostly male medical students was, and still is, a difficult subject. No woman wants a pelvic examination but reluctantly presents to the gynaecologist if necessary, with the same acquiescence as she goes to the dentist; she hopes that the professional can help sort out and cure the problem. To add a second, not quite so skilful, vaginal assessment to the first one is an imposition. Women agreed to it, however, for they wanted to see the best gynaecologists, which meant going to a teaching hospital; this in turn meant medical students. The more altruistic patients would think of those benefits to future generations of women of having doctors properly trained in diagnostic techniques. Alec Bourne was very sensitive to this and considered that one case examined properly was of much greater value to a student than any number of examinations without supervision.[7] Nixon, one of these students, noted this practical sensitivity and took it with him all his professional teaching life.

There were only eighteen gynaecological beds at St. Mary's Teaching Hospital when Nixon was there and so experience was limited. He took maximum advantage of the experiences he could gain, as gynaecology (dealing with diseases of the female genital tract) was usually bonded with obstetrics (dealing with childbirth) to make one focused specialty; in this specialty, Nixon applied himself to both aspects but the obstetric component always remained his first love.

After having completed the full gambit of medical studies, qualification loomed. In 1927, there were three ways of qualifying as a doctor in the United Kingdom. The first was by taking the Diploma of Medicine and Surgery of the Honourable Society of Apothecaries (LMSSA). This was mostly a diploma for students who had studied overseas and British students thought it to be not so prestigious as the other methods of qualifying. The second was by passing the examination held by the Conjoint Board of the Royal Colleges of Surgeons and Physicians (the Royal College of Obstetricians and Gynaecologists did not exist at this time). The diploma given was a Membership of the Royal College of Surgeons (MRCS) and a Licentiate of the Royal College of Physicians (LRCP); this was perceived by many to be an easier examination than the third method, which was to take the London University Final Examination of Bachelor of Medicine and Surgery (MBBS). The Conjoint Examination, however, gave a diploma which allowed young doctors to practise straight away (there were no compulsory house jobs then) but the university degree was required if the candidate wished to go further in medicine, taking the higher degrees of the university such as PhD, MD or MS. However, because of the points in the year at which the examinations were held, by getting the Conjoint Diploma many students were able to qualify a few months ahead of their colleagues who were confining themselves to taking the university examination. In these days house physician and house surgeon posts in the hospital came up every month and not in two clusters in February and August as happens now. So, by jumping the qualification queue, bright people could get a better choice of house jobs and they could always take the MBBS examination later. This is just what Nixon did.

CHAPTER THREE

Postgraduate Training (1927–1934)

Young men know nothing of this sort,
Observant old men know it well.

Why Should Not Old Men Be Mad? (1939)
WB Yeats

Having qualified with the Conjoint Boards Diploma in 1927 at the age of 24 years, Nixon obtained a house surgeon post with Warren Low, by now Senior Surgeon to the hospital and a man of great distinction. He was a Vice President of the Royal College of Surgeons and a President of the Royal Society of Medicine a little later. His position as a surgeon was high but, even more important to Nixon, his influence among his colleagues was very useful for later backing in promotion. Warren Low was a hard taskmaster but he had found William Nixon a self-reliant and reliable student and so was happy to help him with his further education as a house surgeon on the wards. Nixon served in this post until 1928 and started to perfect his surgical skills. At this time, he also worked with Zachary Cope, another luminary in the world of London surgery. Cope always lived close to his work, in this case in Baker Street, so he saw a lot of the out-of-hours hospital life and noted the house surgeons' behaviour. In addition to praising Nixon's surgical skills, Zachary Cope noted, "... he was always kind to patients and tactful in dealing with difficult situations".[1] These were the qualities that would be enhanced later in William Nixon's life.

From here, Nixon proceeded to a house surgeon's post at the Hospital for Sick Children in Great Ormond Street in London for six months. In those days, the best way to learn how to manage newborn babies was to be a house surgeon rather than a house physician. As well as learning about children's diseases, he made his first friends among the paediatric community. He worked for Twistington Higgins, an eccentric but gifted urologist. William returned to St. Mary's Hospital as a gynaecological and obstetrical resident to Alec Bourne and after another six months in 1931 as Resident Medical Officer to Queen Charlotte's Maternity Hospital. While in this post, he had his first two scientific papers published. The first was in *The Lancet* on 'The effect of calcium therapy on toxaemias of pregnancy.[2] Other researchers had shown a

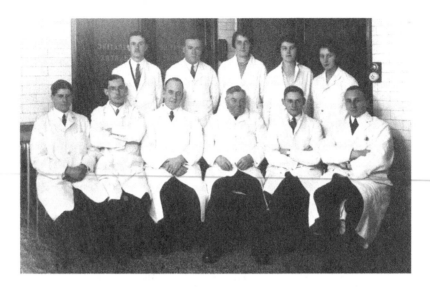

Mr Warren Low (4th from left, front row) and his surgical team at St. Mary's Hospital (1928). WCW Nixon, the junior house surgeon, is on the left at the end of the front row

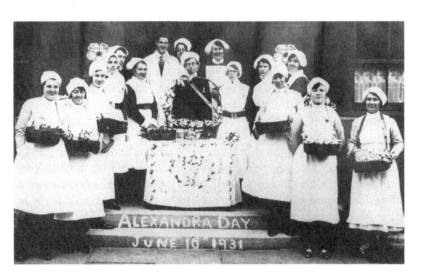

WCW Nixon was a resident surgical officer (equivalent to a junior registrar) at the Soho Hospital for Women in 1931. He is standing over matron's shoulder at the apex of nurses collecting for a charity

reduction in calcium levels in the serum of those with eclampsia and severe pre-eclampsia. Nixon did not confirm this in ten women treated at Queen Charlotte's Hospital; further intravenous calcium glucamate given was disappointing as a treatment and Nixon concluded "... the fits are not influenced by the calcium content of the serum". This was a bold paper going against the stream of scientific thought.

The second paper was of an entirely different nature, 'On the influence of age on labour'.[3] He examined the notes of a hundred mature women aged over 40 years when having their first baby, who had delivered at Queen Charlotte's Hospital over the previous decade, comparing them with a hundred consecutive similar primiparae aged 20–25 years. The eclampsia rates and premature labours were greatly increased in the older group. Infant mortality also was higher in these babies of older mothers while the maternal mortality was also increased (4% *cf* 0%). Nixon concluded that there were risks to the mother over 40 years of age but that death was mostly from toxaemia and this could have been prevented by adequate, skilled antenatal care. The infant problems, he concluded, could have been reduced by a wider, judicious use of caesarean section. He wisely pointed out that most of these older women were never going to have another pregnancy, so surgical deliveries would not be a problem in the future. This paper, although based on small numbers, shows a greater maturity than would be expected of a house surgeon.

He went on in 1931 to be Resident Surgical Officer at the Soho Hospital for Women, a gynaecological unit associated with the Middlesex Hospital, where he worked for Sidney Forsdike, who had a high estimate of his capabilities. Nixon returned as obstetric and gynaecological registrar to St. Mary's Hospital later that year when he was twenty-seven. This post he held until 1933 and it was during this appointment that Nixon showed remarkable foresight and enterprise.

Nixon realised that most of the medical students were going into general practice and that a major aspect of their work would be advising on contraception. In the 1930s, the only methods in use were avoidance of intercourse at the time of expected ovulation (the 'safe period') or the mechanical blocking devices (condoms for the men and diaphragms or caps for the women). However, students had no instruction on these potentially important methods and would arrive in practice less knowledgeable than the women who consulted them. Dr Helena Wright, a pioneer of family planning, recalled receiving a letter from Nixon, a registrar at St Mary's Hospital Medical School, asking if he could bring small parties of his medical students from

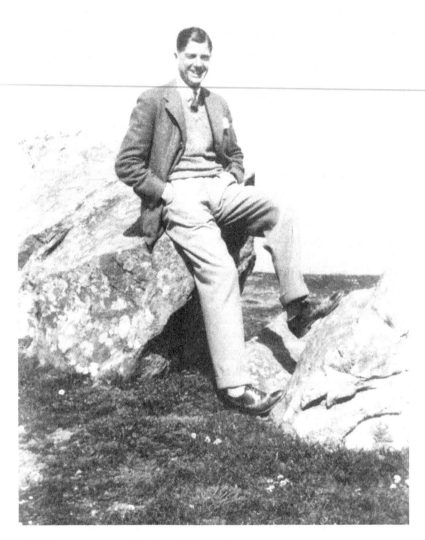

WCW Nixon on holiday in the Scilly Isles (1931)

time to time to the North Kensington clinic to be taught about the theoretical and practical aspects of contraception.[4] After discussion, it was agreed. Nixon and six students would attend of an evening. "He had better bring them on foot, after dark, because they couldn't be seen coming to a birth control clinic in daylight." They arrived before the time of the session to have a technical lecture describing the methods in detail. Dr Wright recalls, "Again and again, Mr. Nixon sat listening to the same lecture, always apparently showing the same interest". After this, the students would join in the practical clinic of cap and diaphragm fitting "… each patient [was asked] if she minded a male medical student watching how her kind of cap was chosen and fitted. The students, although shy, caused the patients no embarrassment".[4] Thus, Nixon saw a problem and dealt with it himself even though he was still in a junior position in the medical hierarchy.

Nixon became the radium registrar of St. Mary's Hospital, dealing with women with gynaecological cancers, and then obstetric registrar to Queen Charlotte's Maternity Hospital until 1935. During this registrarship at Queen Charlotte's Hospital he was invited to prepare a review on menstruation and its association with disease, for the extremely conservative, establishment medical journal, *The Practitioner*.[5] In this, Nixon traced what was known about the relationship of menstruation to systemic diseases. He included work that was then new in endocrinology. He emphasised the whole woman and stressed the need to "use holistic medicine", an early appearance of that adjective in the subject. Although use of 'holistic' in the sense of treating the whole person became fashionable in the last decade of the twentieth century, the idea has been held by thoughtful doctors for many years. Nixon was showing himself to be one of these.

In all these positions he rubbed shoulders with the mighty of obstetrics, who formed the elite consultant staff at Queen Charlotte's Maternity Hospital. He made friends with Leonard Colebrook, the pathologist in charge of Queen Charlotte's Isolation Unit, who later was the first to offer sulphonamides to save the lives of women with puerperal sepsis. Alec Bourne remained Nixon's sponsor. At the beginning of 1931, Nixon was made a Fellow by examination of the Royal College of Surgeons of England. He not only took his MBBS in 1932 but proceeded to the higher degree of MD of the University of London, in which he obtained the University Gold Medal in Obstetrics and Gynaecology. In 1933, at the age of thirty, he became a member by examination of the three-year-old British College of Obstetricians and Gynaecologists.

In the middle of all this clinical and academic activity, William Nixon, who was thirty, now found time to woo and win his wife. A notice appeared in The Times:

"NIXON: YSEBRAND – on February 19th 1934, quietly,
William Nixon MD FRCS, of 14 Devonshire Street, only
son of Professor William Nixon of the University of Malta
and Mrs Nixon, to Miss Vroukje (Vennie) Ysebrand,
daughter of the late Mr & Mrs Hendrick Ysebrand of the
Hague, Holland, and Durban, South Africa".

Vennie was a quiet woman who had been a noted pianist and was a direct descendant of the celebrated early sixteenth-century Flemish artist, Adrien Ysenbrandt. Unfortunately, she had broken her wrist while ice-skating with William and had suffered several unsuccessful operations attempting to reset it; the wrist was never able to stand the strain of concert performances again. William had met Vennie through a mutual friend, Peggy Bradshaw, in the early 1930s when she was studying at the Royal College of Music. They married and had two daughters; the younger, Joy, died of leukaemia at the age of four years; the other was Wendie. To these, William Nixon was a great father; he enjoyed being with his daughters in the times that he could get away from his increasingly heavy workload.[6]

CHAPTER FOUR

Consultancies: at Home and Away
(1935–1939)

Imitate him if you dare,
World besotted traveller, he
Served human liberty.

Epitaph on Jonathan Swift (1931)
WB Yeats

The path to consultancy in the early 1930s was a steep and hard one. Most students, after qualifying, became general practitioners, many joining family practices established by their fathers. A few went into the armed services and even fewer into academic medicine. The remainder (about one-fifth) took the steep and stony road towards becoming a specialist working in a hospital. The forward way for these students involved postgraduate examinations at the universities and Royal Colleges while gaining experience by taking expanding responsibility for patient care in posts of increasing seniority in specialist hospitals. The bastions of these were the teaching hospitals of London and some of the provincial universities. William Nixon had taken all the right steps: he had been a house surgeon to powerful men, he had worked in paediatric surgery, then in increasingly senior posts in obstetrics to the satisfaction of people like Alec Bourne at St. Mary's and at Queen Charlotte's Hospital. He worked in gynaecology at the Samaritan and Soho hospitals, coming back as a registrar for some years at his own teaching hospital.

In consequence, in 1934, when he was thirty-one, he applied for and was appointed as the second surgeon to the outpatients in obstetrics and gynaecology at St. Mary's Hospital. In those days, surgeons were divided into those who had inpatient facilities with the right to admit patients to beds and those who did not. The former were the 'cocks of the walk', the latter were a slightly lesser breed who were hoping the cocks would fall off the perch to make space for them to become inpatient surgeons in time. The difference was not quite so marked in obstetrics as it was in general surgery or gynaecology. In these disciplines, all patients who wanted major treatments had to be

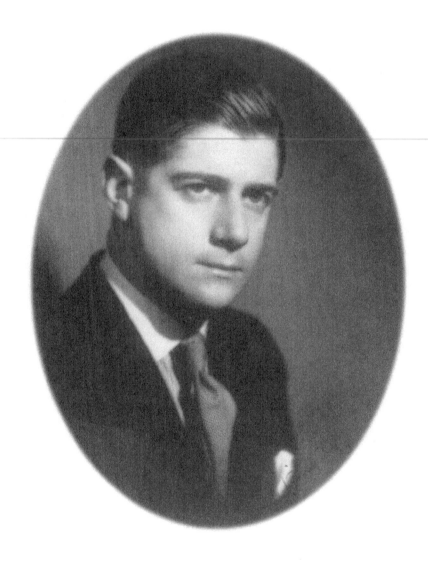

**WCW Nixon in his first year of consultancy (1934). This was the year he married
Vennie on February 19th**

admitted to a hospital bed and therefore would have to be under the name of an inpatient surgeon or physician. In obstetrics, most antenatal work was done in the outpatient departments, with few patients being admitted electively until they came in during labour as non-elective patients. Hence, the difference here between inpatient and outpatient appointments was less emphasised. Gynaecology was rather like general surgery and anyone who wanted to operate on women needed to use the inpatient facilities. There was usually goodwill between the two grades of consultants, with the inpatient surgeons often lending beds to the outpatient ones.

Shortly after becoming outpatient surgeon to St. Mary's Hospital, William Nixon was also appointed in 1935 to the same post at Queen Charlotte's Maternity Hospital, where he performed similar duties. He also saw private patients in Harley Street. He was not entirely happy with his lot; although he loved having the chance to be responsible for women on his own, the situation with private patients was not to his liking. At about this time he noted that the other obstetricians of St. Mary's Hospital were not very old. Alec Bourne, Douglas McLeod and Leslie Williams were in the middle of their professional lives and there might not be a vacancy for a full inpatient surgeon for some time. In consequence, he sought around for advice and it was probably VB Green-Armytage who finally moved him; "Go East, young man" was his advice. Green-Armytage, by now at the Hammersmith Hospital, had been for many years the foremost British gynaecological surgeon in India. He had worked in the whole spectrum of operative gynaecology in Calcutta but was particularly interested in the correction of infertility. He used to do enormously long operating lists in the cool of the morning and also in the evening, with consultations in the middle of the day. He had probably performed more operations than any other gynaecologist. It is said that when Green-Armytage left India, a procession of grateful patients and their husbands half-a-mile long accompanied him to the boat.

William Nixon sought to follow Green-Armytage's advice. He applied for and was appointed to the post of professor in Hong Kong in 1935, a chair endowed by the Rockefeller Foundation that carried with it a consultancy in obstetrics and gynaecology to the Hong Kong government. He and Vennie sailed from England on 12th July 1935, when he was thirty-one. They called in at Malta to see Will's parents and took some weeks to get to Hong Kong.

Although Nixon was welcomed by many of the university staff, he was not universally approved. He met some opposition and obstruction not only from conservative and religious groups in the Colony but also some of his own

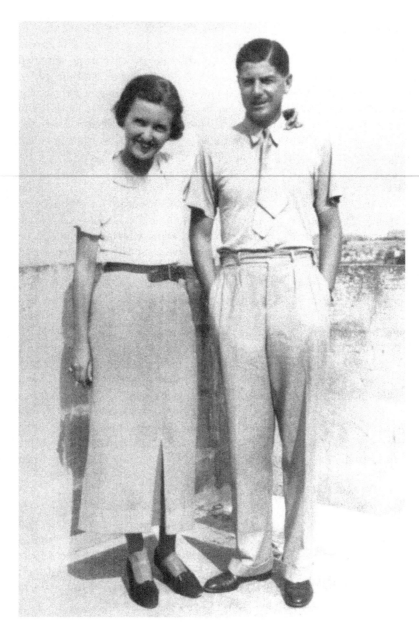

WCW Nixon with Vennie in Malta (1935)

colleagues from the university. He was in sympathy with many of the precepts of Chinese philosophy and he used to try to inculcate aspects of them into his students: the maintenance of an open mind, a humane nature, as well as the application of science for the needs of the human race. He was unswayed by ideas of race, nationality or religion. He met opposition at the old Government Civil Hospital at Sai Yin Pun, over his first operation, which was a hysterotomy, opening the uterus under general anaesthesia for medical reasons to terminate the pregnancy of a woman who was four months (sixteen weeks) pregnant. This was accompanied by tying off the tubes, so preventing future pregnancies. This shocked the operating theatre sister and her nurses as well as many others in that hospital. However, Will Nixon had his principles; there were good grounds for stopping this pregnancy and others, so he operated.[1]

Nixon was much taken with the history of medicine in China and would often refer to it in his later teaching. The Emperor Shen Nung ruled in 2838BC, when we in Britain had not yet even thought of building Stonehenge, which did not come until a millennium later. Shen Nung wrote a treatise on medicine on the effects of diet on the body; he compiled the first pharmacopoeia, which remained the basis of Chinese medicine for several centuries. Diet was considered a very important feature in the maintenance of health and this was exactly in line with what Nixon thought about women in pregnancy. The manifestations of diet deficiency were recognised and described in writings then. Beri-beri, a deficiency of vitamin B1, was described in the fourth century AD. Even when Nixon arrived in Hong Kong in the 1930s, beri-beri was still common. He introduced the use of incompletely milled rice into the diet of the Tsan Yuk Hospital patients. Since this does not have its husk removed, vitamin B1 is still a rich constituent. There was much opposition, not just from the patients but members of the nursing staff and comments were made about "the cruelty of making women take their rice in such an unpalatable form".[1]

Western doctors had to compete with the Chinese superstitions that were still prevalent. Outside the hospital gates were fortune-tellers who sat in booths around the entrance. Nixon used to tell of one mother who would not speak to anyone on the staff after delivery. After much persuasion from one of his assistants, the woman pointed out that the fortune-teller had told her that either she or her child would die on the sixth day after birth. To Nixon's horror both mother and baby died on that very day.[2]

Many other myths were not as serious as this; a simple way of telling the sex of a future child was: "Ask the mother in what month she became pregnant and multiply by the number of the said month. Deduct the number of the mother's age and add 19. If the child is male the number will be odd, if the child is female the number will be even".

This superstition had a sting in its tail. If, according to the calculation, the child should be male but turned out to be a girl "she will surely die at the age of three or five".[2] Until recently, the attendance of male practitioners for women in labour had been forbidden. Only in the last resort was a doctor called and then usually a foreign one, for the Chinese in those days hated a man who attended a delivery and considered him "very dirty and a low person".[2]

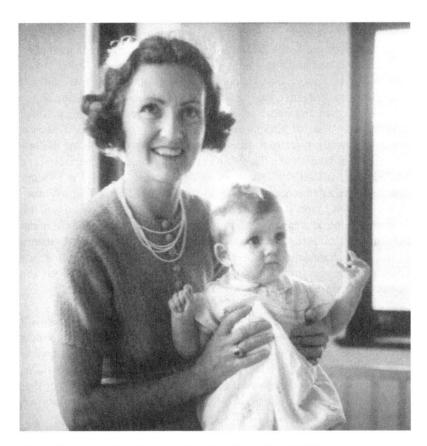

Vennie Nixon with their daughter Wendie in Hong Kong (1937)

The students that Nixon taught in Hong Kong were undoubtedly very fortunate and the few now alive still talk about his work as the best teaching they ever had. He used to give lectures without notes which the students found clear and precise; they were illustrated for emphasis with appropriate stories at the right moment. His clinical rounds in Tsan Yuk Hospital were always fully attended. He used to separate the fifth- and sixth-year students into two groups which he called the sheep and the goats. The sheep were the final year students being prepared for the slaughter of the impending qualifying examination. They were placed in the front row of the group on the ward round and each member had to answer a series of questions in turn.[1] This was good practice.

While in Hong Kong, William Nixon made a point of meeting as many Chinese people as he could. Being a man of great sensitivity and gentleness, he appreciated these same qualities shown to him by other people. He was greatly impressed by the intelligence of those he met, their propensity for hard work, their culture and their respect for knowledge and learning. He also admired their cheerfulness, their love of life and their hospitality. The European community as a whole, both business and Service, kept itself aloof from the Chinese, meeting only in common interests of horse racing and dining.

He was made a Member of the Hong Kong Medical Association and of the Chinese Medical Association and he used to love to attend the meetings. At such an occasion, on 5th May 1936, William Nixon gave an address on postpartum haemorrhage.[3] He started with a plea for gentle conservative management of the third stage but included reports of basic research work on ergometrine by John Chassar-Moir back in London only six months before. He pointed out that violation of the gentle principles of placental delivery was the most common cause of postpartum haemorrhage. He outlined treatment as it was then, with emphasis that the medical attendant should stay with the mother for at least half an hour after placental delivery, a wise precaution. Later that year he sent a report back to Britain of a lithopaedian.[4] This is a rare mass formed in the uterus when a baby dies before birth but which is retained and slowly fibroses then ossifies, its presence often only being diagnosed many years later.

When Nixon arrived in Hong Kong, the perinatal mortality rate (stillbirths and early neonatal deaths) was 300 per 1000 births and families of ten children were not uncommon. Nixon, knowing these two were linked and following his principles, set up the first family planning clinics and took his medical students to them. This shocked many of his colleagues but luckily he had Professor Lindsay Ride, the Principal of the University and later its Vice Chancellor, on his side. The beginnings of the family planning movement a little later in mainland China may well have stemmed from what Nixon did in Hong Kong. He insisted that students were taught about this valuable aspect of health care and although the methods used then were rather more simple and mechanical than now, he managed to persuade many women in Hong Kong to have smaller families. This was against the tide of popular opinion, which sought to provide as many children as possible to care for the parents when they reached old age.

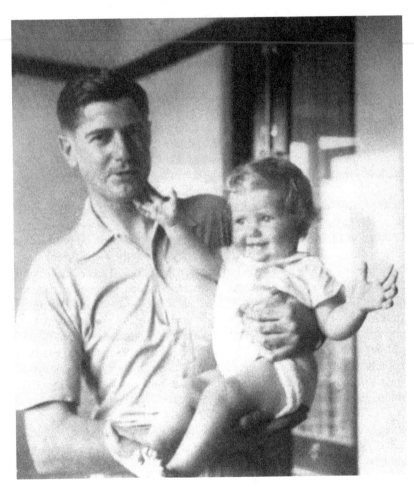

WCW Nixon with his daughter Wendie in Hong Kong (1938)

Nixon's research in Hong Kong was mainly obstetric-based. He surveyed oedema with the help of funding from the Ella Sach Plotz Foundation, writing up the results in the *Chinese Medical Journal*, to which he submitted a review on oedema in pregnancy.[5] This thorough review of the subject is notable for being written through the experience of Hong Kong. Although some of the references are of European and American origin, most of the article referred to the Chinese population he treated and paid attention to the effects of malnutrition. A fuller account of this subject also appeared in the *Journal of Obstetrics and Gynaecology of the British Empire* with a similar title.[6] Here, Nixon repeats his clinical observations but offers fuller treatment regimens.

Nixon also sent back to the *British Medical Journal* an article based on his Hong Kong experience of 'Aids in the diagnosis and treatment of ectopic gestation.[7] In it, he emphasised the need for a carefully taken history and clinical examination, especially looking for pulsation in the fornix of the vagina of the affected side. This was elicited by allowing the tip of the index finger of the vaginal examining hand to "… rest gently on the region of the attachment of the vagina to the cervix" to feel this palpation. Culdocyesis with a needle (entering the pouch of Douglas from the vagina into the lower peritoneal cavity) is a valuable test and a full laparotomy should be performed if there was any doubt. He also stressed the usefulness of autotransfusion of blood, from the peritoneal cavity back into the woman's circulation, another forward-looking idea in the contemporary surgical scene, when blood was a valuable commodity.

In 1938, the Japanese army had advanced well into China, taking Tsingtao, Canton and Hankow. They had installed a puppet Chinese government in Nanking and had withdrawn from the League of Nations. Their forces were moving south on the eastern littoral of China. By this time, William and Vennie were both very concerned about the future of the colony in relation to the Japanese invasion. Nixon felt that his work in Hong Kong was done and he returned to the United Kingdom in early 1938. He left many good friends behind and even more students whom he had taught. They would come into his life again and again when he returned to London and were always welcomed. Nixon left with goodwill from the people of Hong Kong where he had endeared himself to the residents by his "mannerisms, characteristics and famous phrases".[1]

Vennie and their daughter travelled back by boat ahead of Nixon, taking the long route and calling in at South Africa on the way for a holiday to see her brother and his family, who lived in the Durban area. They all returned to live in London at Rivermead Court in Putney next to the Hurlingham Club and

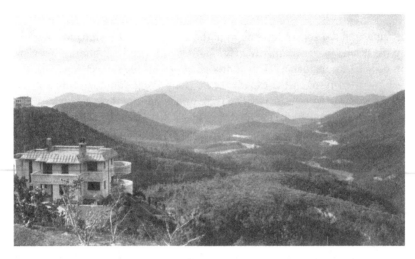

The house on the Peak, Hong Kong, where WCW Nixon and Vennie lived while he was professor at the University (1938)

Wendie went to a nursery school nearby. While awaiting another appointment, Nixon continued to write up his experiences from the Professorship in Hong Kong. A review of the diagnosis and treatment of disproportion appeared in *The Practitioner*.[8] Nixon, however, welcomed the recently published work of Caldwell and Moloy,[9] who had subjected a large number of pregnant and labouring women to stereoscopic X-rays in order to elucidate the effects of pelvic size and shape on performance at delivery. Such studies would not be done now but in 1938 the effects of irradiation on mother or fetus were not considered serious and so this work was performed by doctors, unaware of any potential harm. In his review, Nixon stressed again conservatism and patience in awaiting results of long labour. "The dislike and fear of the Chinese (attributable to Confucian doctrines) for any sort of mutilation by operation forced one to temper judgement with conservatism and to adopt a less radical attitude towards obstetrics than is practised in the West."[8] This lesson permeated Nixon's professional life.

Also as a result of working in Hong Kong, Nixon published a short article on endometriosis of the bladder.[10] This rare condition usually needed surgery to cure and he published this article as a warning to doctors who dismissed female urinary symptoms too readily with a bottle of alkaline mixture and no attempt to make a diagnosis.

William Nixon had been invited to share a platform with RA McCance on 11th May 1938 at a course on maternity and child welfare in London. McCance was a well-known nutritionist in the Medical Research Council's Biomedical Research Unit at King's College Hospital, London, and became famous at the end of the Second World War for his work with Belsen victims. Both speakers stressed the need for a first-class diet in pregnancy and the teaching of the elements of nutrition to women. Nixon detailed the clinical manifestations of diet deficiency and his contribution shows the way he was already thinking for practical use later.[11]

Will Nixon was appointed a consultant in 1938 to the Soho Hospital for Women, the gynaecological wing of the Middlesex Hospital, a large teaching hospital. On the staff were many experienced and well-known gynaecological surgeons and here he was able to perfect further his techniques of surgery, which led him into the top flight. There were some who tried to contend that Nixon was not a good operator. On the contrary: there are reports from many who watched his surgery who were amazed at his dexterity and ability to tease out surgical problems with the minimum of blood loss or infection after the operation.

CHAPTER FIVE

The War Years (1939–1945)

And therefore I have sailed the seas and come
To the holy city of Byzantium

Sailing to Byzantium (1927)
WB Yeats

When the war started in September 1939 Will Nixon was thirty-five. He was exempted by the authorities from military service as his civilian work as an obstetrician and gynaecologist was too valuable. At the Soho Hospital for Women he was put in charge also of the emergency casualty unit, a part of the Emergency Medical Services (EMS) of London, to deal with those injured in air raids on the capital. This was at its maximum load in the winter of 1940/41. During the Blitz one of the worst episodes that Nixon had to cope with was the bombing of the Café de Paris in the spring of 1940. This smart nightclub was crowded with four hundred people when it was attacked. Fourteen were killed and over one hundred injured by the glass ceiling falling in. The Soho Hospital was just up the road from the club and Nixon took much of the strain of medical work. Will Nixon was able to cope with this, doing much of the work himself and allocating the rest to various grades of more junior doctors. He also took more than his share of the rota of fire watching on the hospital roof, detecting and dealing with incendiary bombs, which would often follow the dropping of high explosives. The Soho Hospital was not damaged greatly, no doubt partly thanks to the efforts of the firewatchers.

As well as the Soho Hospital, Nixon had been appointed a Consultant in Obstetrics and Gynaecology at St. Mary Abbott's and Paddington Hospitals, both run by the local authority, London County Council. The load for a consultant in all three of these hospitals was increased, as numbers of junior staff were reduced by the needs of the armed services. However, many women had been evacuated from London at the beginning of the War and during the Blitz. Nixon and others were kept there in case of need, but he had time to think about his researches. He published a paper in the *British Medical Journal* about the excretion of vitamin B1 in toxaemia, showing that the amount of the vitamin was less in the urine and placental tissues of those with a normal pregnancy.[1] The study was notable by its inclusion of patients not just from London hospitals but also from Glasgow and Sheffield. Multicentre studies were unusual in those days.

Two invitations in these early war years gave Nixon a chance to refine his ideas on the effects of nutrition on pregnancy. He was invited by the Council of the Royal College of Obstetricians and Gynaecologists to give its most prestigious annual lecture in October 1941: the William Blair Bell Memorial Lecture, in memory of the College's founder. He chose to speak on diet in pregnancy and was able to lay out his ideas on this with further opportunity of a long printed account in the College's journal.[2] This encapsulated Nixon's thoughts and should be read by anyone interested in this subject. A second chance to consider his thoughts about nutrition followed an invitation from the *British Medical Bulletin*. Here, he reviewed studies done (including an excellent bibliography) and practical steps for the improvement of maternal nutrition.[3]

Nixon was very worried about his wife and children being in London during the air raids. He repeatedly tried to persuade Vennie to go to her family in South Africa. At first she resisted but eventually Nixon started to make bookings on ships sailing out to South Africa. Vennie's response was to cancel these but, in time, very reluctantly, she agreed and she and the two girls departed in convoy. They sailed to Durban where life was easier but she still worried about Nixon. In Durban, the youngest daughter died of leukaemia at the age of four, leaving only Wendie.[4]

Meanwhile in London, Nixon, parted from his wife, met a woman with whom he became enamoured. Sidonie Marcus (Sidi), an Austrian refugee from the Germans, was working as a biochemist at the London School of Hygiene and Tropical Medicine and at St. Mary's Hospital in London. She had escaped from Vienna with the help of a British journalist. By the end of the War, the relationship between Sidi and Nixon had flourished considerably.

Meanwhile, there was a strange episode in Nixon's life. He had been asked by the British Council in the middle of the conflict to go out to Istanbul to be their medical representative. This would be associated with a Chair at the University. At that time, Turkey was teetering on the brink of joining the Axis of Germany and Italy against the Allies. The Foreign Office was involved in this exchange and Nixon, a great patriot, went out at the age of forty, in the middle of the war, to fly the flag for Britain.

The Governors of Soho Hospital for Women released him for the duration and after some slightly complicated manoeuvring at the Foreign Office, Nixon sailed through the Mediterranean in December 1943. The attempted air and sea blockade by the Axis powers had eased by now. The worst attacks on shipping were in 1942 but the Allied landings in Sicily in July 1943 caused the reduction of available Axis airfields; while the sea threat from submarines and Italian warships remained for a while, the need there had been for attacking Malta had faded.

Nixon went first to Egypt in convoy to Port Said. He spent two weeks in Cairo, where he was hospitably received by Professor Naguib Pasha Mahfouz, one of the great Egyptian gynaecologists, who had a fine international reputation. Mahfouz dealt particularly with vesicovaginal fistulas where damage had led to a hole between the bladder and the vagina. In consequence, an uncontrollable leak of urine flowed from the vagina. The women were always wet and smelled of urine so they soon became outcasts. Such damage was often a result of long labours and the birth practices in Egypt; Mahfouz was highly successful in their repair. Nixon spent every day of his two weeks watching him operate either at the Coptic Hospital or the Fouad I Hospital. By this time Mahfouz had gynaecological experience that was unrivalled. Dealing with the damage caused by the crudities of obstetrics and gynaecology formed the bulk of his practice. He had a special ward of ten beds devoted to women with vesicovaginal fistulas and his museum would have been the answer to a pathologist's prayer. There were three floors devoted entirely to obstetric and gynaecological pathology, all the items beautifully illustrated, photographed and catalogued. Mahfouz himself was a fine artist who used to draw the operating specimens, positioning them back into their site in the body to give an air of verisimilitude. Nixon loved this short visit and would have stayed longer sitting at the feet of Mahfouz but had to get on to his real destination.[7]

Nixon completed his journey to Ankara by car and train up through the Taurus mountains and on arrival in Turkey was met by his compatriots, who immediately took him out to Karpitch Lokanti, a Russian restaurant and a rendezvous of all nationalities. It was the centre of fashionable life and Nixon was fascinated to see the crowded dance floor and the clientele, often in national military uniforms of armies who were engaged in fighting each other in other parts of the world. A diplomatic armistice was observed in the restaurant and crowded dance floor and Nixon warmed to its strange food and wine and the beautiful women.

It was a tonic after drab, war-torn London. William Nixon departed for Istanbul and he well remembered the enormously congested night express, with its crowds of peasants in their colourful clothes who seemed to be carrying with them all their belongings including mattresses. Army officers in jackboots and civilians of all classes carried flowers, fruits and sweets.[7] The congestion on board was enormous. They travelled through the night and reached Hayadarpasha, the terminal of the Baghdad railway, on the Asian side of the Bosphorus. From here, Nixon had to travel by ferry across the water and for the first time saw the dove-grey and olive-green domes and walls of Byzantium that is now Istanbul. He saw it many times later from the Bosphorus, but his first impression of that dawn always stayed with him. He was put up in a hotel, which was then in rich woodland just outside the town but with a good bus and train service to the centre.[8]

Stories of what William Nixon did in Turkey vary and none can now be substantiated, despite application to both the Foreign Office and the British Council for the release of documents. Perhaps the papers are still not in the public domain, held back by the hundred-year release rule. There is a record of one letter in the minutes of the governors of the Soho hospital on 2nd July 1940 from Lord Lloyd, President of the British Council. He asked that Nixon be released from the Soho Hospital to undertake work of national importance and that he be promised reinstatement on his return from Turkey.

There are those who emphasised his major influence as that of a great teacher and scientist trying to make the medical intelligentsia of Turkey appreciate pro-British ideas. Others said that he was a member of the British Intelligence Service, there to counter the efforts of the British Ambassador's valet, Cicero, and the German Ambassador, Von Papen, a pair of spies. One source even said he put out counter-intelligence that was instrumental in leading the Germans to keep regiments of troops, who were badly needed at the Russian front, in the Middle East. Apparently, Nixon is supposed to have started the idea that two divisions of the Indian Army were poised to pass up through Persia and invade Turkey, the 'soft underbelly' of Europe.

There is a view held by Nixon's family that he was used by British Intelligence. He left a series of diaries in code about his Turkish adventure but unfortunately these have not survived to the present day. He also told several people (including Elliot Phillip) that when he retired to Malta, he would write his biography, which would not just be about his obstetric and gynaecological career, but "my life as a spy".

Not even in the height of the War would an agent be sent to a foreign station with its many different languages, cultures and religions, without some training. There is evidence in the hospital minutes that Nixon took eight months off from his hospital work in London (February to October 1942). In that time, basic instruction could have been given about specific matters. An Inter-service Balkan Intelligence Centre had been set up in Istanbul in December 1939 for the collection of information and later for recruitment, training and running disinformation agents in the Eastern Mediterranean.[9] The personnel obviously, were mainly natives of Turkey, Syria, Palestine and Egypt for a European would have stood out when covert work was required. These agents and some double agents were mostly used to start misinformation filtering through to the Germans to give the impression of even stronger Allied forces on the Syrian and Turkish borders, but London enlisted personnel could have been used for specialist missions.

Wendie McWatters, his daughter, went to Istanbul in 2003 to meet with Professor Aykut Kazancigil, the current Professor of Obstetrics at the University.[10] His father had held that position in 1944 and knew Nixon well – indeed, was responsible for getting him to Turkey. They became close friends and Nixon spent many happy weekends at the family beach house on the Marmara Sea. The current Professor Kazancigil, as a boy, used to enjoy swimming with Nixon and taking him out in his boat at weekends.

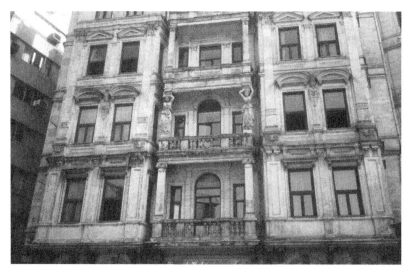

The Grand Hotel de Londres, Istanbul as it is today. WCW Nixon lived there for his stay in Turkey (taken by Wendie McWatters 2003)

Apparently, the Turkish Government offered many German Jewish exiles key academic posts at Istanbul University. Professor Kazancigil considered that Nixon had been dispatched by the British Intelligence to blend with the Jewish expatriates, establishing contacts and getting secrets from them. Many had families still inside Germany and it was felt that the Jewish doctors would have no sentimental attachment to the Third Reich. This German Jewish community at the university refused to speak anything but their native language. Nixon's mother was half German and Nixon spoke German well. Could it have been brushed up in London between June1940 and December 1942?

William Nixon had a suite at the Grand Hotel de Londres, opposite the Pera-Palas Hotel – a notorious rendezvous of international spies. Nixon was there often and he also used to dine frequently at Rejans, a Russian restaurant famed for its blinis and exchange of secrets. It is obvious that Nixon could not have afforded to stay in such an expensive art-nouveau hotel on his salary had he not been subsidised. The Garbara-Capo school of Medicine still exists and the office used by Nixon is still occupied.

William Nixon was a great patriot and would have used his position at the university to propagate anything that would have harmed the enemy. The wives of many politicians and high-ranking army officers came to him professionally because of his reputation and so he met many who influenced policies and he made sure that they learned the British point of view.

In an excellent review of Nixon's life, Professor Richard Beard, an obstetrician who later trained with Nixon at University College Hospital, recounts a strange incident.[11] He tells of an attempt made by Nixon's pro-German first assistant to undermine his position in 1944. At the end of one hard operation in Istanbul, while closing the abdomen, the theatre sister leant over and whispered to Nixon that she had been ordered by his pro-German colleague to discredit him as a surgeon by infecting the wound of his patient with dust from the theatre floor. There is no other record of these assertions but it is just the sort of thing Nixon would have relished, as indeed he would have any form of adventure.

Each day, Nixon would go to work in the hospital on public transport and get off a short distance from the clinic so that he could walk over the Galatia Bridge towards the Golden Horn, passing the Hippodrome, the aqueducts and many other sixteenth-century buildings. On arrival at the clinic at about eight o'clock, he would change into a cool white shirt and slacks and shake hands with the assistants and sisters who were already assembled. He would then

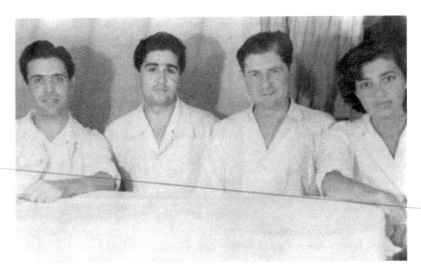

WCW Nixon (3rd from the left) with his surgical team in Istanbul (1944)

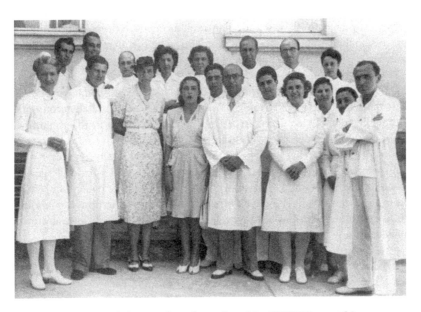

Lady Peterson, wife of the British Ambassador, visits WCW Nixon at his department in the University of Istanbul. WCW Nixon is second from the left, standing in the front row

drink a cup of Turkish coffee and a glass of iced water before starting work. This began with systematic lecturing to audiences of up to four hundred students, with latecomers sitting on the floor and window ledges and crowded around the rostrum. Nixon had as an assistant a very good interpreter, who had been educated at the American Girls' College and could translate as the lecture went along, thus avoiding the business of written translations. She also went on his ward rounds, which must have been amazing, as they were conducted in a hotchpotch of English, French, German and Turkish. At the end of the ordeal of the lecture and ward round, more coffee was served and then outpatients or operating sessions would start.

Nixon took his turn on the rota of being on call as consultant for night emergencies. During each duty week he slept in his office, feeding on Turkish food with the junior doctors. He considered that he learned much about the Turkish way of life in this way and in the cool of the evening he would walk through the cobbled streets of the Tartar quarter. His clinical work consisted of dealing with fistulas of all sorts, growths of the pelvic organs, inflammations, osteomalacia and congenital abnormalities. He considered that the Turkish peritoneum had "an extraordinary natural immunity – one could get away with all kinds of assaults on it".[8]

Both antenatal and postnatal clinics were run efficiently and, in gynaecology, a fertility clinic was started by Nixon. This was very popular as, in a Muslim country, a woman who cannot bear children can be divorced very easily. In such fertility sessions, he insisted on examining the husband as well and remembered one who was very annoyed, having brought his three wives along because none of them had borne children. Tests showed that it was the man who was suffering from a very low sperm count; his three wives were gynaecologically normal. The man left the clinic in a rage, his wives trailing after him, no doubt smiling behind their yashmaks.

Among other honours, Nixon was made a Member of the Turkish Obstetrical Association and used to take part in its Higher Examinations. This he remembered well and he thought that they were constructed in a more intelligent way than the British ones. In brief, the candidates would present themselves after three years of residency work, with their prepared thesis on some aspects of obstetrics or gynaecology. If this was accepted, a practical examination followed. This took the form of a clinical examination, an oral test and an operation performed on a patient under anaesthesia in front of the examiners. The three examiners then put forward three questions to the candidate who picked one of them and went away to write for an hour on the subject. If this answer was considered to be satisfactory, the candidate was dispatched to the Ministry of Health, where he was given a diploma and a certification number to use for prescription purposes.

A man of Nixon's personality made friends very readily and he enjoyed greatly the social life of Istanbul. He received and gave hospitality, enjoying the Turkish food, and many good friends were made who would come to see him in future years when he returned to London. There is one particular episode for which Nixon was especially remembered in Turkey. He swam the Bosphorus. This is a major waterway draining from the Black Sea into the Sea of Marmara and thence to the Mediterranean. It is nineteen miles long and varies in width from two and a half miles to nine hundred yards at its narrowest. It divides Europe from Asia and splits Istanbul in two. When William Nixon was there, no bridges had been built across the Bosphorus (the first being constructed in 1973) and the only way across was by ferryboat. The Black Sea was a closed body of water into which drained the major rivers of Eastern Europe – the Danube, the Diiestr and the Don. The only outlet was the Bosphorus, with its thirty-metre decline of the seabed from north to south.

Surface currents flowed mostly from north to south. There were, however, two layers of water, the upper a freshwater flow on the surface, with a lower counter-

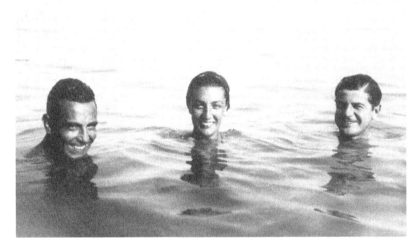

WCW Nixon swimming in the Bosphorus with Pierre Eumroze, his principal assistant, and Mrs Eumroze (1945)

current of saline water from the Mediterranean, itself an enormous, tideless, almost landlocked sea. These two flows did not mix and with the variations of width in the straits led to dangerous swirling currents, which were exacerbated by local sea winds, causing vortices and even whirlpools. The rate of the upper current might have been relatively slow on the surface but this was speeded up by variations of the seabed, especially in shallower waters.

All this made the strait dangerous for swimmers but it has challenged the romantic through the ages. Io, the goddess later named Isis in Ancient Egypt, swam it. So did King Dorian and later Lord Byron, who both swam the longer route across the Hellespont; hence, the attraction for the romantic Nixon to try, for he was a powerful swimmer. He crossed from the area of Rumeli Hisar, just above the narrowest point where a four-knot current would have been running at that time of year. Later in the winter this can be seven knots, an unswimmable force. The distance directly is just under a mile but the oblique course to benefit from local currents was close on three times that.

We are lucky to have Nixon's own account of this in the *UCH Gazette:*[8]

"I had heard of some of my compatriots swimming the Bosphorus but had not met any of them. I knew that the narrowest crossing was at Rumeli Hisar, the fort on the European shore built by Mehemmed the Conqueror in 1452 to cut off supplies and possible relief for Constantinople from the sea. There was a strong current from the Black Sea to the Marmora, which a naval friend estimated at about four knots. He calculated where I should land on the Asiatic shore. I decided to train seriously for the attempt. It was now autumn and the sea still delightfully warm on the Marmora side, but several degrees cooler in the Bosphorus. Preparations for my departure [for the UK] took much time during the last few weeks and gave me ample excuse for not attempting the swim. I realised I was making these a form of escape. Time passed and I found I had only 24 hours before leaving for Ankara – still I procrastinated. What was to be gained by swimming from Europe to Asia and trying to emulate in lesser degree Byron's feat of swimming the Dardanelles? I must decide either to continue with my packing or drive by taxi to Rumeli Hisar. I chose the latter and changed into my bathing trunks while in the taxi. The driver looking askance and when I alighted threatened to call the police. But after telling him I was one of those mad Englishmen he quite understood.

A Greek fisherman was luckily close by who agreed to take my clothes and row close to me. Having reached this point what use was it to put a toe in the water to see if it were cold? I plunged in and tried to swim towards a point directly opposite but the current was too strong and I was soon drifting westwards. The Greek was a great help by pointing to the mark on the Asiatic shore towards which I still tried to swim. My naval friend had warned me of the danger of shipping. I had not seen any ship when I entered the sea, but by the time I was half across a 10,000-ton ship from the Black Sea was bearing down on me. She obviously would not deviate from her course and was travelling at about 10 knots. I knew I would be disappointed if I stopped now and clambered into the boat. As she approached my position I could see she was an American Liberty ship. The captain seemed to appreciate my position and after three blasts of the ship's siren graciously turned to port.

There were no other incidents until I reached the Asiatic shore. It was difficult to get a grip on the rocks and while trying to pull myself up a small barnacle buried itself in the pulp of my little finger. I paid off the Greek fisherman and found myself in the garden of a private house. A Turkish lady came out of the house and in perfect English invited me to take tea. I asked her why she spoke English to me and she replied that only an Englishman enjoys such futile heroics. By now my finger was painful and I was relieved to meet her husband, an ex-naval surgeon who had studied in England. After some coaxing, the barnacle was extracted. Tea and Turkish cognac revived me and I was exhilarated in the achievement of having swum from Europe to Asia."

This incident led to many stories. It was put about that the young lady who received him was very beautiful and had entertained him well for three days and nights. This is unlikely in view of the fact that her husband was busy operating on Nixon's finger at the time. However, Dennis Hawkins, one of Nixon's lecturers later at University College Hospital, referred to an occasion twenty years later in 1966 when a still-beautiful Turkish lady turned up at UCH wanting to see the Professor.[12] He was found, remembered this woman and entertained her royally in London, telling his students she was the woman who had looked after him on arrival from the Bosphorus into Asia.

During this time his father, the former Professor of Mathematics at the University of Malta, had moved back to England and, while Nixon was still in Turkey, had died. Since the War was on, Nixon was unable to return to see his father or to get back for the funeral. He had been very fond of his father, who had inspired him to go on in academic life. Nixon's mother was also in London by now and Nixon wrote to his uncle, Dr John Hobart Nixon of Chippenham, to ensure that his mother was being looked after.[13] Relations with Vennie, who was still in South Africa, were distant. When the War in Europe finished in May 1945, Nixon's task in Istanbul seemed to be finished. He made a prolonged round of friends, all of whom appreciated the work he had done for Turkish women, his teaching of obstetrics and the practice of it. His stay in Turkey was profitable also for an important paper[14] on icterus in pregnancy, in which he and his Turkish colleagues sorted out the confusion in the classification of jaundice in pregnancy. He made it clear.

In the autumn of that year Nixon, now forty-two, came back to Britain to the Soho Hospital, from which he had been allowed special leave to go to Istanbul. Soon, however, the Chair at the University College Hospital Medical School became vacant. Nixon applied for it with Bourne's backing and was appointed in 1946.

CHAPTER SIX

The Obstetric Unit in Nixon's Time
(1946–1966)

We and the labouring world are passing by:
Amid men's souls, that waver and give place
Like the pale waters in their wintery race.

Rose of the World (1892)
WB Yeats

When William Nixon joined University College Hospital as Professor in Obstetrics and Gynaecology, he took over from Professor FJ Browne, the first incumbent at that academic unit. Just after the First World War, the Rockefeller Foundation had made a bequest to UCH with the aim of establishing units that would help the development of medical education. Medical and surgical units were started in 1920, with funds provided for teaching on a scientific basis. The department of obstetrics had to await the building of the new Obstetrical Hospital next to the UCH site and so it was not until 1926 that FJ Browne was appointed a Professor of Obstetric Medicine. He took up his first duty of reorganising and improving of the teaching of obstetrics and gynaecology by strengthening his current staff to provide for this.

Browne held antenatal and postnatal clinics in the hospital, which he and his staff attended with the first aim of teaching medical students. Gynaecological patients were shared for teaching purposes between the members of the academic unit and the honorary staff, of which there was only one consultant at this time – Clifford White. With the completion of the new Obstetric Hospital, the number of women attending for delivery increased rapidly. By 1929, one-third of the women having babies in the Borough of St. Pancras did so at UCH and many more were admitted from outside the boundaries. Until that time, there had been joint wards for the nursing of maternity and gynaecological cases but, to avoid the risks of cross-infection, Professor Browne divided these up and also started a small isolation ward for cases with suspicion of infection.

Browne was lucky to attract Chassar-Moir, who came from Edinburgh and worked as research assistant at UCH until 1935 when he moved across to the Postgraduate Medical School at Hammersmith, eventually becoming Nuffield Professor in Obstetrics in Oxford. While at UCH, Chassar-Moir performed major research work on ergometrine, the stimulant of uterine muscle contractions. Physiologists and pharmacologists were not convinced by the anecdotal accounts of obstetricians that the contractions of the uterus in response to this drug were stronger than any other oxytocic agents. Chassar-Moir set out to provide objective evidence with the help of Dr Davies, then Chief Pharmacist at UCH, who made the special extracts used in the experiments. This was done in the labour wards, then on the fifth floor of the Obstetric Hospital at UCH, using a balloon filled with mercury placed in the uterine cavity after delivery and connected to a pressure recording system, which in those days was a rotating carbon-smoked drum with a sensitive stylus tracing a white line on the drum paper. The selected drug was injected into the mother and the pressure rise produced by the contractions of the myometrium recorded. The effect of various oxytocic drugs could thus be compared semi-quantitatively. Women, however, were sensitive to the presence of the drums with their moving traces in the room, so Chassar-Moir led a tube out through the window and along a ledge into the next room where the recording equipment was kept. This worked well until the pigeons of Gower Street,

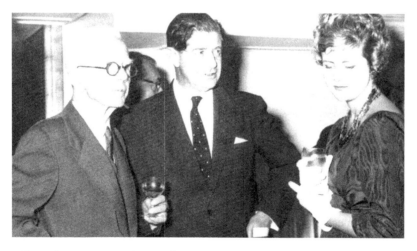

WCW Nixon at a reception in the Savoy Hotel with his predecessor, Professor F J Browne and Will's daughter, Wendie (1958)

finding the red rubber a fine flavour, started pecking at the tubing, thus releasing the mercury and invalidating pressure records. The solution was to drill a hole in an internal wall and pass the tubing through it into the next room.

In 1934, Browne's title was changed. He had held the Chair of Obstetric Medicine; now it was more properly named Chair of Obstetrics and Gynaecology. He had already appointed Max Rosenheim as a research worker in the field of hypertension in pregnancy. Rosenheim, as a medical student at UCH before the antibiotic days, had researched and developed the use of mandelic acid for treating urinary infections, a massive problem. He went on to be a professor of medicine at UCH and was eventually created Lord Rosenheim, President of the Royal College of Physicians.

One of FJ Browne's major teaching interests was antenatal care. He established teaching clinics in this discipline, recognising the antenatal period as a time to detect and prevent problems that would impinge on labour. This was the first of the multiphasic screening systems. Browne started the first London Flying Squad in obstetrics at UCH in the 1930s, (the original idea for a squad was from Newcastle); anaesthetists and specialist obstetricians could be sent immediately with all equipment pre-sterilised and packed in heavy metal drums to help women in their homes. Later a small (too small) second-hand car was bought by Nixon's department funds, painted in UCH colours and used to carry staff and equipment. When Professor Browne retired from UCH in 1946 he went on to Australia, where he continued his work on pre-eclampsia and antenatal care for many years. He left at UCH a unit that was a model for many others.

Nixon's assistants at UCH

Nixon was fortunate to inherit assistants of some seniority and much talent. The first was Aileen Dickens, a strong woman with marked views on teaching and training for overseas doctors. She lived in a Regency house just off the Edgware Road and was a tower of strength for Nixon, supporting him in hospital committee tactics in his early days. Dickens was a consummate medical politician who later became vice- president of the Royal College of Obstetricians and Gynaecologists. One of the other assistants was Josephine Barnes (later Dame), a highly qualified doctor who worked and talked hard, a good operator, allegedly capable of performing a caesarean section in four minutes from incision to skin stitch while complaining good-naturedly about the slowness of her operating attendants. She was liked by the students as her teaching was dogmatic and she had personality. She used to drive around London very fast in sports cars and had a reputation for never being late for an outpatient clinic or an operation. From UCH, she joined the Charing Cross Hospital as a consultant and later was President in turn of both the Medical Women's Federation and the British Medical Association. Jo Barnes was in much demand for Royal Commissions; for example, on the working of the Abortion Act, on assisted fertility and on medical education, as she spoke much sense, pithily and to the point. Another assistant was Gladys Dodds, a fierce, little woman who got her own way in most debates. She left after a few years to go to a chair in Hong Kong. Richard Buckell, a registrar who later went on to be a consultant in Poole, completed the team.

Gerald Swyer was appointed in 1947 as a research assistant in endocrinology and became a consultant three years later. A man of many parts, he made models and musical instruments in his spare time and enjoyed dinghy sailing. He outstayed Nixon, retiring only in 1978. He started, with Nixon, a fertility clinic at UCH, which he himself used to call a "futility clinic" because of the infrequency of successful results. Swyer's contribution to hormone endocrinology was well known and, at UCH, began many of the basic science investigations of sex hormones. These are considered in Chapter 7.

In 1947, Fouracre Barnes was also made an assistant; he was a man of great strength and took a particular interest in diabetes in pregnancy, a neglected condition until that time. He had plenty of ideas and died too young, at forty-two. Nixon was very fond of Fouracre Barnes but that did not stop him from stepping in if he thought something was not right. For a short while, Fouracre Barnes started to use stilboestrol in early pregnancy in an effort to try to prevent miscarriages. Much later, this was shown to be a harmful drug causing abnormalities of the fetal genital track and, later, vaginal malignancy. Nixon had disapproved strongly of its use long before this was known. However, fortuitously, most women did not attend the clinics until well after the phase of pregnancy when it may have been useful (about eight to twelve weeks of gestation), so it was not a widely used drug. Nixon persuaded Fouracre Barnes of the potential dangers of these ideas and this therapy was discontinued at UCH. Unfortunately, in the USA, the use of stilboestrol persisted and led to a mini-epidemic of malignant and premalignant cervical and vaginal disease.

In 1948, the team assisting Nixon changed to include Jack Dumoulin. He had been parachuted into the Balkans in the War and returned to medicine afterwards, taking higher training in obstetrics. Dumoulin had a nice, barely suppressed sense of humour and all the students loved him for it. While Aileen Dickens was on study leave in Copenhagen for six months, Dumoulin was made first assistant and Elliot Philipp, a clever worker with interests in the fertility field, filled his locum. Philipp went on to become a tower of strength to the National Birthday Trust for thirty years.

Nixon also managed to attract from general surgical work, a research assistant in obstetric anaesthesia. Dr Shila Ransôm was the first real obstetric anaesthetist in London. She was responsible for much work on pain relief in labour and in gynaecology, introducing regional spinal anaesthesia for operations and epidural anaesthesia for childbirth. She took an active role in the antenatal teaching of women so that they knew what to expect in labour. This was an important part of Nixon's philosophy. In a similar vein, he established an obstetric physiotherapy department. Helen Herdsmann was the first to staff it. Although she only stayed a short while, it was she who started to help pregnant women learn and practise correct exercises. She was followed by Helen Hylton-Jones. The physiologist, Helen Payling-Wright, came to the UCH unit and did much research for many years on blood flow in the veins of the leg, blood clotting and the effects of labour and pregnancy on these processes.

In 1948, Mavis Gunther was seconded by the Medical Research Council and, while not a paid member of the unit, she was given full accommodation and facilities. She was particularly knowledgeable about breastfeeding. While there had been a clinic for women who had problems with breastfeeding started by FJ Browne, the work now expanded enormously to involve all women who delivered at UCH. Mavis Gunther used to go round the women each day talking to them about breastfeeding and breast problems. She was known, perhaps irreverently, to many of the students as "The Breast Queen", but her work in her gentle persuasive way was invaluable to the mothers in the days when formula feeding was not very reliable. She helped thousands of babies in the first weeks of their lives and is remembered with affection by women who had their babies at UCH during her reign.

The idea of paediatricians looking after newborn babies was then new but Nixon had great faith and among the first things he did was to put the neonatal nursery entirely under the care of the neonatal paediatricians, a farsighted move by an obstetrician in 1946. He used to hold meetings once a week to discuss problems and WG Specter, the pathologist with a special neonatal interest, usually attended these.

Nixon always gave responsibility to his assistants. He let them proceed with any reasonable management even if he disagreed with it. If anything went wrong he would be there to pick up the pieces without any recriminations. If the assistants did well, he was always first to praise them. Should problems occur, he would talk with them quietly in his office, which in the early days was near the front door of the Obstetrical Hospital. He came into the hospital early in the day and caught up on what had happened overnight. Thus, those who had encountered a problem could talk with him before the day's official work began.

Family planning

Another innovation introduced almost immediately was the establishment of a family planning clinic. UCH was then the only hospital in London to have such a clinic and Nixon was keen that students should attend and learn about this important aspect of life. If not there, where were they going to be taught the necessary techniques that they would need in later practice? Deans and ruling councils of the medical schools in those days were very narrow-minded. They finally agreed to Nixon's request for a family planning clinic but insisted it be held on a Wednesday afternoon – traditionally a free half-day to allow rugby or cricket to be played. In those days, the subject was not discussed in public; the session was known as "the clinic in the Records Department".

As we have seen, when Nixon was a registrar at St. Mary's Hospital he had arranged to go with a small group of students after dark to the North Kensington Family Planning Clinic which was near his hospital. He had taken the idea to Hong Kong and had even started such a clinic when he was in Istanbul, in a Muslim country. When he came to UCH, he continued to believe in the importance of family planning (still mostly condoms and caps, although Nixon himself favoured the Graafanberg Ring). Joan Mallison, who he invited to start the first contraceptive clinic in a London teaching hospital in 1949, helped him in this endeavour. From this, the needs of women led to the start of a session in psychosexual problems. In 1955, Joan Mallison died; Sylvia Dawkins and Barbara Law took over. They persuaded Michael Baliunt, the psychiatrist, to join and help train doctors deal with psychosexual problems. From this early beginning came the Institute of Psychosexual Medicine. Barbara Law remembers how she and Sylvia Dawkins lectured on the subject and allied psychosexual problems. Later, they were allowed on to the wards as well, to see women before they went home. Nixon catalysed the making of a film about the clinic in action and another on sex education called 'Learning to Live'. He started a trend in the use of films by medical people to help teach the public.[1]

The Queen Bee

The Queen Bee of any obstetric unit is the labour ward superintendent. The Matron or Senior Nurse may outrank her in the nursing hierarchy but the labour ward superintendent has most influence on the medical staff and

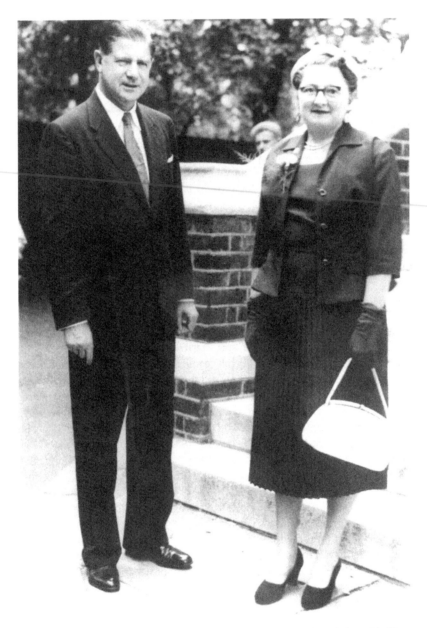

WCW Nixon and Sister Billings at Dennis Hawkins wedding (1955) (provided by
Professor Dennis Hawkins)

midwives. At UCH during most of Nixon's time she was Sister Margaret Billings ("Sister Bill"). She ruled the labour ward, the powerhouse of the Obstetric Hospital, controlling midwives, students, junior doctors, and often seniors too, with a vocative rod of iron. When Nixon first arrived they were at daggers drawn but Sister Bill soon succumbed to his charm. Having rebuked a staff midwife for some misdemeanour outside the door of a labour ward, Sister Bill could turn the door handle, go in and be all sympathy for a mother within whose labour was taking longer than expected by all, especially the woman herself. It was also said in UCH that Dr Shila Ransôm was responsible for reforming this tough labour ward superintendent, who was really a midwife with compassion and thoughtfulness for women in labour. Certainly, Bill enjoyed a drink with male company when off duty; all the registrars and assistants would ensure to bring back a bottle of good malt whiskey when returning from overseas visits. The love of her life was Hughie, a marine engineer with one leg. He visited UCH when on leave in London and eventually they married after Bill's retirement.

Part-time consultants

Making use of all the skills he could, Nixon felt that work in research and teaching should not just be in the hands of the academic staff. There were also part-time doctors in the hospital who were both in private practice in Harley Street and giving their time to the hospital, for there was no salary for consultants before the National Health Service came in, their appointments being honorary. When Nixon arrived at UCH there was only one part-time consultant gynaecologist, Clifford White, who had been at the hospital for many years. He was a gentle, quiet man but very persuasive and the students liked him. White had a pungent wit, which many students remembered all their lives. Once he asked a student, "What would you do with a case of severe postpartum haemorrhage?". The answer came back, "Give morphine". White commented, "Well, I suppose that would just about give you time to get to the coast".[2]

Soon after Nixon's arrival, White was joined in 1948 by Tim Flew who was more rumbustious and always ready to give an opinion full of sound sense but also full of wit and good teaching. These two started the practice of part-time consultants working hard alongside the academic unit and not in rivalry to it. Flew was a short man of rapid words and good with his hands in theatre. His ward rounds were humorous and much appreciated by the students but, most importantly, they remembered what he taught. He stayed as consultant until the 1960s and was a great supporter of Nixon. Later, for four years, Flew was part-time Dean of the Medical School. In that position he always had an eye to help the academic department in the Obstetric Hospital. He was still in post when Nixon died. He was joined by Jo Holmes, more a straight man, who was a first-rate surgeon and when he taught, the students could understand what he had to say.

Antenatal care

The antenatal clinics were expanded and women were seen by all members of staff, usually accompanied by students. Nixon recognised that the antenatal clinic was a marvellous place where students could, in the course of a morning, see a large number of women with a great variety of conditions, each of which could act as a text for a short sermon by himself or a senior member of staff. It did mean that the women might have to wait and so the large waiting hall of the antenatal clinic was expanded.

Nixon invited members of the Women's Voluntary Service to start a cookery demonstration stand in one raised corner of the hall. Rationing was still in force until the early 1950s in Britain and Nixon used the idea of cookery classes to proselytise his ideas about diet in pregnancy. Tasty recipes were prepared with the basic foodstuffs that were available and among this advice were the subtle lessons of nutrition in pregnancy such as the value of the skin of a jacket potato. This had been usually discarded, but Nixon knew that most of the nutritional vitamin and mineral value lay just under the skin. Similarly, his time in Hong Kong had shown Nixon the nutritional value of the Chinese style of cooking. He tried to introduce this to the diet at UCH but was too far ahead of his time and the management would not accept it. The food from the outpatient demonstrations was usually consumed by the women (and any medical students who were lurking at the edges of the crowd). This was a very good practical method of putting his nutritional ideas over, as well as passing the time waiting to be seen in clinic.

In another corner of the hall was a screened-off area where physiotherapy suitable for various stages of pregnancy was taught and practised. Nixon, having agreed with Grantly Dick-Read about the psychosomatics of pregnancy and pain relief in labour, found willing allies in the physiotherapists who ran this aspect of antenatal care and propagated it. In addition, husbands were made welcome at these classes; this was a great innovation. It did the men good to gain some practical understanding of their wife's problems during pregnancy; it was also found to be helpful in the labour later: it was Nixon who opened the labour wards to fathers in the 1940s.

Further staff changes

The staff was strengthened by the arrival of John Martin. He was from St. Thomas' Hospital in London. He has described how, at Lewis's bookshop in

1950, he met a friend who was at that time the resident obstetrician at UCH.[3] They had gone to have lunch in the pub opposite the Obstetrical Hospital, which is now called The Jeremy Bentham. Martin was told that UCH was looking for an assistant for the obstetric unit and as he said, "Next, I found myself in an office with Will Nixon, who was asking me about my research interests". He was selected and started work in March 1950. Since he was not very experienced in gynaecological surgery, Jack Dumoulin, the senior assistant, took him under his wing. Martin describes how work at UCH was an eye-opener, as there were women doctors on the staff. In his previous post at St. Thomas' Hospital, there had been none. There was a general opposition to women at this time from the higher reaches of medicine and John Martin relates that at St. Thomas' Hospital the opposition to female medical students was based on the grounds that there were not enough women's lavatories, despite the fact that over a thousand nurses worked comfortably in the hospital.

Martin returned to St. Thomas' in 1954 but came back in to UCH as first assistant in 1959 for two years. He was the workhorse of the department, nearly always on duty, but he regretted the time when he was not able to do research. He did, however, take part in one very far-reaching piece of work with Jack Dumoulin on giving prophylactic ergometrine after delivery to prevent postpartum bleeding of the mother. This is considered in the next chapter.

John Martin also reports taking part in an exercise, literally, which Nixon had ordered, which emphasised his enthusiasm for antenatal physiotherapy. All the male medical staff were told to attend the physiotherapy department in loose-fitting clothing, in order to experience at first-hand the rigours of antenatal gymnastics. John reports how idiotic they felt putting their thighs and legs in the air while the chief physiotherapist, Helen Herdsmann, urged them to bear down. An off-duty house surgeon, exempt from the class and passing by, looked through the door and retreated, his face contorted with mirth. He reported to the rest of the Obstetrical Hospital the terrible sights that he had seen.[3]

Nixon continued his recognition of the place of therapeutic abortion, no doubt following his mentor, Alec Bourne. Probably more abortions were performed in UCH during this time than at any other teaching hospital in London.[3] This was before the Abortion Act 1967 but covered by the *Ober Dictum* made in the Rex v Bourne case (1938). John Martin finished his time at UCH in 1959, after he had stood in as Deputy Director when Will Nixon went to Ceylon and India at the behest of the World Health Organization. Martin was subsequently appointed to a senior post in Perth, which led to his becoming Professor there.

In 1954, Josephine Barnes was appointed a consultant at Charing Cross Hospital and left UCH, while Pells Cocks, who had been resident assistant obstetrician for two years, went down to Bridgend as the first consultant obstetrician. He had been greatly influenced by Nixon and so the new department was built on Nixonian principles. Thus it stayed for the 26 years that Pells Cocks was in charge. Richard Law replaced him at UCH as resident assistant and went on to take other posts in the unit. He was a great devotee of Nixon as he saw the human side of the man. For example, Nixon suggested to Law that he should go to the Centre International de l'Enfance in Paris (he was a fluent French speaker) for six months on a scholarship. Nixon found the

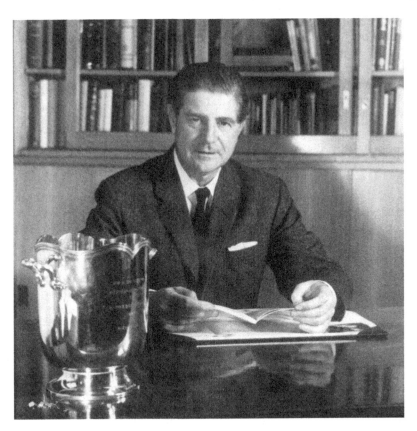

WCW Nixon in his office at UCH with the Owen Geffen Rose Bowl awarded to his unit for its institutional care of mothers and babies (1957)

time to write a long handwritten letter to him there, giving the UCH gossip and keeping him in touch with home. Law was a popular teacher who made himself expert at vaginal breech delivery. He later took up a consultant post at the Whittington Hospital and so stayed within the gambit of UCH. Norman Morris became first academic assistant. Morris was a man truly in tune with William Nixon. He believed passionately in the woman's right to take a major part in her own labour. He was already involved in the psychological aspects of the subject and his time at UCH allowed him to expand this to become a lifelong interest. He later became professor at Charing Cross Hospital.

An influential visitor to UCH was Grantly Dick-Read. Will Nixon had always agreed with the ideas of this doctor, who considered women's feelings in labour and worked with antenatal education to try to prevent pain in labour. A woman who knew what to expect was more relaxed. This, Dick-Read believed, reduced the pain and length of labour. Once, as a junior doctor in Whitechapel, he had witnessed a normal delivery and a woman had refused a chloroform mask to relieve labour pains. Afterwards, when asked by Dick-Read why, she replied, "It did not hurt. It wasn't meant to, was it doctor?". He established a school of thought that many less forward-looking obstetricians refused to adopt but William Nixon became a faithful devotee. When the National Health Service was introduced, Grantly Dick-Read disagreed with it furiously and he left the country to work in South Africa. In the mid-1950s, at Nixon's invitation, he came back to UCH to lecture on preparation for childbirth. Dick-Read used this it as a reason to drive up the length of the African Continent over six months, studying the birth practices of many tribes on the way.

Norman Smyth became a Nuffield research assistant and he added enormously to the weight of research into fetal heart activity in labour and uterine action, (discussed in the next chapter). Dr Cicely Williams, famous for her work on nutrition in West Africa, was made an honorary member of the Unit and worked there on infant weight gain. She had first described kwashiorkor and malnutrition in Ghana and championed breastfeeding rather than powdered milk feeding, a potentially dangerous practice when clean water was difficult to get.

Outside interests

Professor Nixon did not like committees, but if he thought it was worthwhile being a member, he pulled his weight. He served for twenty years on the UCH Medical Committee from 2nd October 1946 to 2nd February 1966, being chairman for part of that time. In 1955, Nixon was elected to the Council of

The Royal College of Obstetricians and Gynaecologists, representing London obstetricians. He attended regularly the Saturday morning meetings each year for six further years, in roles varying from monitoring the research obstetrician's post at the Medical Research Council Unit in Oxford, to speaking wittily and sharply at the Annual General Dinner in 1957. He represented the RCOG in international affairs as the expert adviser on maternal and child welfare at the World Health Organization. As well as this, he served on many committees of the RCOG, such as that with the British Paediatric Association, giving freely of his time and expertise.[4]

Nixon was, at this time, also on the Council of the Royal College of Midwives and a member of the politically influential Standing Maternity Committee of the Ministry of Health. It was that year that the National Baby Welfare Council awarded the Owen Geffen Rose Bowl to the Obstetrical Hospital and the Infant Welfare Department for the best institutional care of mothers and babies. The Director was also nominated as the University representative to the Medical School Council at St. Mary's Hospital, a position he greatly appreciated, having spent his early days there. He was also appointed to the Management Committee of the Institute of Obstetrics and Gynaecology at Queen Charlotte's Hospital.

Nixon was honoured by being made a foreign member of the Gynaecological Society of Uruguay. The friendships that William Nixon had started overseas were coming back to roost. Visitors were being sent by their governments from Turkey and Hong Kong, as well as USA and South America. Nixon was appointed to a working party of the Medical Research Council to investigate the problems of congenital abnormalities.

It is interesting that some who worked in the UCH Obstetric Unit at this time considered that there was a dichotomy between the research workers and the clinical workers. The former did not have to attend meetings and apparently did very little teaching, while the latter did the hard work of both the clinical department and the teaching load. Ill feeling could have grown between the two groups but Nixon saw to it that it did not break the surface nor become a permanent feature. A staff improvement that Nixon negotiated was for reasonable duty hours for his junior staff. At UCH in the mid-1950s some senior consultants were "insisting that their own house officer (the most junior grade of doctor) be available twenty-four hours a day, seven days as week". One of the author's friends, Philip Fulford, only had one weekend off in six months and that was because his consultant's wife said that "Philip looked tired". (Fulford came to no long-term harm from this, becoming an orthopaedic surgeon, a Commander in the Royal Navy and the Queen's Surgeon on the

Royal Yacht, Britannia.) Not wishing to grind his staff into the ground, Nixon insisted that they had one evening off in three and one weekend in three. If he caught the junior doctor still on the wards on one of the evenings he was supposed to be off duty, he would chase the offender away.[3]

Secretaries

One of the most important positions in UCH Obstetric Department was the Director's personal secretary. When Nixon first arrived, Miss Rita Wanklin, who had been FJ Brown's secretary for many years, was still in post. She left in 1952 and was replaced by Nancy Champion, who got on well with her boss, whom she thought of as "kindest, wisest and most generous of men, giving tirelessly of his skills and time". He took to heart the troubles of many who called on him and worked hard to help them. Miss Champion left in 1959 to get married and was replaced by Mary Alexander, Nixon's last personal secretary. She ran his professional life with great efficiency, always trying to save him from unnecessary fatigue or from doing things that irritated him and made him angry. She was efficient but fair and all outsiders who wanted to approach Nixon had to go through her. Mary's extreme tact included never intruding on the professional relationships between Nixon and his staff. Hawkins remembers her well. "Most of the time she was both authoritative and pleasant but never more than that, and every inch a lady, always immaculately made up and immaculately dressed."

After Nixon's death, Mary Alexander joined the administrative staff of the Royal College of Obstetricians and Gynaecologists. She became, in turn, head of the Examination Department and is still remembered there as a fair leader, always insisting on discipline among the (mostly) female members of staff who ran that most important department. They all had to dress neatly, uniformly and moderately. It was Mary Alexander who made a point of meeting overseas doctors who had come to Britain to take the Membership Examination (MRCOG). These men and women were often confused and frightened but Mary Alexander was kindness itself to this group of obstetricians. Sometimes she was the major contact they had in the RCOG structure and they remember her still in many parts of the world.

Major projects

After a couple of years of mulling over ideas, in the mid-1950s William Nixon was beginning to put into fruition his plans for a national survey of births. This started as an idea to compare home and hospital deliveries as, in those days, about one-third of deliveries were at home and two-thirds were in hospital. He spent some time gathering his co-operators and fundraising bodies. This idea turned into the famous National Perinatal Mortality Survey, which is described more fully in Chapter 7. It involved so much work that he eventually allocated one member of staff, Dennis Bonham, his first assistant, to look after the obstetric side of it. Both Dennis and Nancie Bonham spent many hours analysing the enormous amounts of data generated. Nixon was fortunate in getting Neville Butler, a UCH paediatrician, to supervise the paediatric aspects. Albert Claireaux, the pathologist at Queen Charlotte's Hospital, managed the pathology.

This was also the time of the beginning of another of Nixon's big ideas; a special unit for research into mother and child problems began with the Nuffield Research Team in 1955. The professor, Norman Smyth, Mrs J Ferrow (a research electrical engineer) and Miss MH Bainbridge were the first researchers, bringing together the instrumentation that had been prepared over the earlier years for measuring various levels and activities of mother and fetus and recording their results on punch cards. Now was the era when statistics became an important aspect of any research study and Nixon saw to it that his unit was well advised and practised in this aspect. The details of the development of this unit also can be found in Chapter 7. It caused great interest in many of the obstetric units in London, Europe and the world. Scientists came to UCH to see what was happening now that William Nixon was enabled to concentrate his research into one area.

Further staff

At the beginning of 1956, Herbert Reiss joined the Unit as an assistant. Reiss did research on cervical incompetence, vaginal hysterectomy and abortion at later gestations. It was he who persuaded Nixon to change from intra-amniotic urea injections for late terminations of pregnancy to the much safer hypertonic saline. He was one of the most loyal of Nixon's staff and was known for his kindly, helpful and considerate manner. The following year, Reiss left to become a senior lecturer in Hong Kong. Pamela Bacon joined the Unit as an Assistant. Nixon visited America, travelling from the West to East Coast, lecturing and making more new friends. He visited many of the major centres and was warmly received.

William MacGregor became first assistant. He was an outward looking, active Australian man who had worked at Bristol and was very keen on teaching. He had an original approach to obstetrics and gynaecology and stimulated his students. The assistants often came to him for advice and never went away empty-handed. Bill moved on to become Reader at the Postgraduate Medical School, Hammersmith, two years later, where he repaid some of the debt he owed Nixon by looking after his daughter in childbirth.

In 1959, Martin had returned from St. Thomas' Hospital as first assistant. He soon had to cover for Nixon, who had been invited to visit Ceylon (Sri Lanka) and India for six months as an adviser to the World Health Organization. Again, it is interesting to note that Nixon's powers of persuasion were used at Colombo University to see if he could bring to an end the feuding between the Tamils and the Singhalese in the medical school there.

To provide senior cover and to enhance the teaching, UCH Medical School invited Alec Bourne to come out of retirement and be a locum consultant at the Obstetric Unit while Nixon was away in Ceylon. He did this willingly, despite having retired from St. Mary's Hospital five years before. It is interesting to read accounts of how people were impressed by Bourne's deft handling of junior staff and by his skills in surgery of the uterus. He had a great feeling for Will Nixon and his Unit, particularly the humanity he found there.

> "I was struck by the modern teaching of human relations under the direction of Professor Nixon. Thus, the pregnant woman realises she should not just be a 'case' but a real human being, as she had been in her home, and the knowledge of modern pain-killing techniques during labour removes so much of her natural fear that for this reason too she will face labour with almost calm indifference and certainly unafraid. Professor Nixon has also created a maternity department renowned for a kindly personal relations between the doctors, midwives and patients are the key to the contented happiness of the patients."[5]

The following year (1960), William Nixon had his first coronary thrombosis (Chapter 10). During his time away, Pamela Bacon covered the clinical load. The Medical School authorities again asked Alec Bourne to come back in a part-time capacity to provide senior support. In the following year, Pam Bacon moved on to become a consultant at the Elizabeth Garrett Hospital and Don Menzies, from Liverpool, was made the first assistant. He was an excellent and experienced obstetrician to whom staff members would turn when in trouble. He put on a tough exterior but really had a soft heart. The story is told by Hawkins of a day in gynaecological outpatients when there had been a discussion going on behind the curtains for five minutes. Don Menzies then emerged and said in a quiet voice, "She's a nice lady with a chronic pelvic inflammation which is slowing resolving. She comes to me every month. Sooner or later the inflammatory disease will have resolved completely. In the meantime, it is only five minutes every month of my time to keep her away from aggressive surgeons".[3]

Hawkins returned from the Postgraduate Medical School in Hammersmith to become an assistant on the Unit. Rudi Saunders joined and introduced the vacuum extractor to the unit. After using it successfully himself for over thirty deliveries, he convinced the Professor of its value and taught the other members of staff to use it.

While Bonham continued refining testing an enzyme method of detecting cervical precancerous changes, he was doing more work on the Perinatal Mortality Survey. This survey was beginning to attract attention around the world and Bonham had invitations to discuss its findings at the National Institutes of Health in US and in Austria.

The study achieved both fame and notoriety: the former because it was the first time that a total population of babies was looked at and their deaths examined; the latter because of the way it was presented to the public and the effect on the workers concerned. Nixon was the man who presented the survey results at press conferences and on the wireless (this was in pre-television days) making dramatic pronouncements about obstetric care, referring to "kitchen-table obstetrics" and "mothers dying unnecessarily". Many felt that this was excessive but not Will Nixon, who was determined that the public should know what was going on and almost sacrificed his reputation with the doctors, but such was his standing that he, too, rose above it. Claireaux was also sufficiently senior for the impact of the Perinatal Mortality Survey to do nothing but good for his reputation. Butler, rather younger, rode above it because he was that sort of man and, being a paediatrician, was only responsible for the babies after the delivery. Bonham was attacked for exposing facts and antagonising the general practitioners; soon afterwards, he went to New Zealand as Postgraduate Professor of Obstetrics at Auckland.

Later years

In 1962, Geoffrey Theobald retired from Bradford and Nixon appointed him to UCH as research fellow. This was a great feather in the cap of the Unit for Theobald was an original thinker. He had been responsible for the shift in philosophy in the use of Syntocin® to stimulate labour. He pioneered the titration of oxytocic stimulation of the uterus by the labouring mother's own response to the length and strength of her uterine contractions, thus individualising treatment and putting it in the hands of the woman herself. Theobald had a great interest in the Royal Navy, having served at the Battle of Jutland in the Great War. While in the Unit he continued his work on the electrical induction of labour,[6] an intriguing concept. After Nixon had died, Denys Fairweather, his successor, made Theobald an honorary senior research assistant. He continued his research but it was overtaken by the great efficacy of the prostaglandins in stimulating labour.

In 1959, a government committee considered the value of mass miniature chest X-rays for antenatal patients. After a survey and an enquiry, this was dropped and those who were at higher risk of tuberculosis had the less hazardous full chest film. UCH was one of the first to abandon this potentially dangerous investigation. The use of X-ray pelvimetry was also examined. The standard three views used in the non-pregnant woman gave the maximum irradiation and so a standing lateral view only was started. Probably, this film alone provided 85% of the useful information contained the older procedure.

William Nixon still took on his mantle of heavy duties, both in and outside the hospital. In addition to examining in several London medical schools and at the Royal College Membership Examination, he still examined at Cambridge. Nixon's unit was continuing to receive visitors from all over the world, many sent by the Ministry of Health, the British Council, the Postgraduate Medical Federation and the World Health Organization.

Anthony Woolf joined as a resident assistant obstetric surgeon. This was strictly an NHS post but the Professor made it quickly clear that a part of his job was the overseeing of the academic unit assistants. He also had the task of bringing up to date the annual reports of the whole department, an obsession with Nixon. This he did, but every time Nixon saw Woolf in the department, he reminded him of the task. This drove Woolf to remind Will Nixon that "only my wife was allowed to nag me".

Don Menzies had been appointed as first assistant with senior registrar status two years before. He was advanced in 1963 to consultant by Nixon. This was apparently to enable him "to perform abortions with less fear of prosecution before the Abortion Bill was passed".[7] The Bill finally reached the House of Commons in 1967 but Nixon had had a large part in its earlier drafting. Not only did he argue for therapeutic abortion, but encouraged its performance at UCH. "I do not think there was another teaching hospital in London at that time frequently undertaking this operation and Nixon was on the forefront of the pro-abortion supporters, no doubt influenced by Alec Bourne."[7] The load was such that Dr Elizabeth Tylden, a wise psychiatrist with great feeling for women inadvertently pregnant, was appointed to the staff of the Obstetric Hospital to help with the problems of termination of pregnancy.

Will Nixon had another coronary thrombosis in 1964 while staying in Brighton. He was taken off duties on each occasion but stayed away too short a time. On his return he was irritable and apprehensive that he might be invalided out of his post. The following year, Kelsey Harrison, himself a graduate of UCH, was seconded from John Lawson's department in Ibadan, Nigeria, for a year's research. On return to his home country he became Professor at Abu Bello University in Northern Nigeria and later Vice Chancellor at Port Harcourt on the coast.

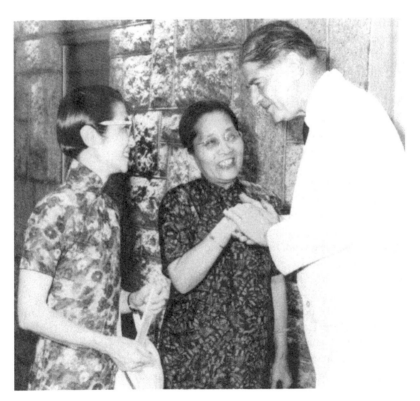

WCW Nixon greeting two old friends during a visit to Hong Kong (1965)

In 1965, PN Suter was appointed as an assistant. He was renowned for his discipline. He had been graded as an obstetric specialist in the Royal Army Medical Corp. Bonham departed for New Zealand having finished his work with Butler in the Perinatal Mortality Survey. William Nixon was invited as visiting professor and external examiner to the Hong Kong University, at the invitation of the Postgraduate Medical Federation. He performed an extensive tour of the academic centres in the Far East in the same visit.

Richard Beard joined the Unit and worked with Theobald. Richard was one of the brightest stars in the young obstetricians' firmament. He went on to be a noted Professor at St. Mary's Hospital, Nixon's old Medical School. He did much to unify European obstetrics in later years. In 1965, Hawkins was appointed Professor at Boston University School of Medicine, USA.

Generally, William Nixon's staff were a happy team. Whenever possible, he tried to appoint people he felt would best fit rather than of necessity select someone with a particular clinical ability. What mattered to him was their personality and ability to get on with the other members of staff.[1] In this he mostly succeeded.

CHAPTER SEVEN

Research at the Obstetric Unit (1946–1956)

All men live in suffering
I know as few can know,
Whether they take the upper road
Or stay content with the low,
Rower bent in his row boat
Or weaver bent at his loom
Horsemen erect upon horseback
Or a child hid in the womb

The Wild Old Wicked Man (1937)
WB Yeats

By the time most research workers reach their fifties, they tend to gravitate towards one of two categories. One group carries its research from previous years well into maturity; this is unusual. Most scientists are in the second, finding that their research efforts are at the best in the years of life between twenty-five and forty-five and after that, their capacities for original thought and unravelling of serendipitous conclusions are lessened. The second sort of senior research worker can still spark ideas from younger people, catalyse them and guide their research. Often, less mature researchers need constant reminding of their aims and objectives and require a mentor to check frequently how their work is going. William Nixon achieved both groups. His later ideas on research would now be considered socio-medical and he kept on pioneering them. However, he was also able to winkle out the best ideas from his juniors and then help them to plan the structure of their research projects from the beginning. He then had the capacity to keep them going by frequent meetings when they had to present what they were doing and what progress had been made.

A monthly meeting for the Co-ordination of Obstetric Research started on 15th November 1948 and continued for the years of Nixon's Directorship. He himself took it very seriously and is recorded as attending three-quarters of meetings where a record was made of those present, quite an achievement considering the Professor's many commitments in teaching, examining and advisory bodies outside the hospital. All senior and later junior staff attended. Any research projects were brought here, discussed and, if agreed, reported on at intervals.

Workers from other research institutes were invited to present their material to the UCH group. A member of the department who went on a study visit to other centres would share briefly their experiences with their UCH stay-at-home colleagues. Requests for samples of maternal and fetal tissues came from workers in UCH, UCL and many other centres. Some priorities had to be set up and the rare times these failed are recorded in the monthly minutes and Professor Nixon was irritated. By this means, no research would go on without all being informed and no group of women was being over-investigated. Formal records were made and approved each meeting by one of the group elected as secretary. These volumes still exist in Professor Charles Rodeck's office and were reread with interest in preparation of this biography.

By this triple approach, Nixon established the UCH Obstetric Unit as a national then an international centre of research, particularly into the physiology of uterine contractions, the biochemistry of the woman in pregnancy and the measurement of various fetal functions while still in the uterus. He helped others with their work on pain relief in labour, blood loss at delivery, more meticulous care of the mother with diabetes and the problems arising from blood clotting. No one who had any good ideas was turned aside by Nixon. He listened to his house surgeons and students, often encouraging them to do research projects on their own ideas with his guidance. He encouraged them to help each other. For example, when one worker was working on uterine muscle contractility, he made everyone who performed a caesarean section remove a small snip of the uterine wall to be kept in oxygenated saline for that research. For about two years, Nixon checked personally that this was done at every caesarean operation to help this one junior research worker.

Endocrinology

Through the researches of Gerald Swyer at UCH Obstetric Unit, much of the endocrinology of gynaecology and obstetrics was disentangled and new managements were proposed. At first, Swyer was a research assistant at UCH, taking over the new laboratory built in place of the old lecture theatre on the top floor of the Obstetric Hospital. His interest was in the metabolism of progesterone in normal and abnormal pregnancies, including those that ended in miscarriage.[1] From the beginning, he cooperated with Fouracre-Barnes in working on the association of low serum progesterone levels to the outcome of the pregnancies of diabetic mothers.[2] At that time, mothers with diabetes either did not get pregnant or commonly lost the pregnancy early on. If the fetus survived after 30 weeks, growth was excessive and led to both maternal and fetal problems in labour; stillbirths were common. Over the years, he extended his techniques to measure oestrogen and gonadotrophins in non-diabetic mothers, separating the two hormones by partition chromatography.

From the beginning, Swyer's research was also helped by Nixon starting special outpatient clinics; one was for the investigation and treatment of infertility[3] and the other for female endocrine diseases. These were swamped by women who wanted help that could not be obtained from any other specialist clinic in London. Work followed on the use of vaginal-wall smears to determine hormone levels in the body. Both oestrogen and progesterone affect the morphology and staining properties of vaginal surface cells. These could be obtained easily by vaginal-wall smears and their microscopic characteristics would give broad clues to the hormonal state. Glucose tolerance studies in pregnancy were initiated. Hormone studies in normal and premature children at the time of puberty commenced and work on giving progesterone to those women at risk of spontaneous miscarriage was continued. Evaluation showed that 85% of women continued their pregnancies and about 10% more than those on more conservative therapy.

In 1951, Gerald Swyer was made a full consultant in endocrinology to University College Hospital but his first love stayed with reproductive medicine and his work was still set in the Obstetric Hospital. The determination of oestrogen levels in body fluids including urine commenced at UCH, one of the two units in the United Kingdom where this was done. This led to the whole Byzantine structure of using oestrogen levels in the mother's urine to estimate fetal and placental function. It became a universal test of fetal wellbeing, coming to an apex in the 1970s but gradually declining after that with the development of more predictive biophysical ultrasound measures of fetal wellbeing.

By the mid-1950s the work of the laboratory had increased in volume so that a technician was required to work full-time on just the routine examinations of obstetric and general hospital patients. Swyer felt this intruded on research and so he squeezed finance out of the hospital for an extra worker. Visitors to the laboratory continued the work to perfect their own special interests. For example, Dr Yucel was seconded from Istanbul University to work on the changes in the cells of vaginal smears in relation to the hormone status of women. He took this work back to Turkey and established a laboratory there, which carried on these investigations.

Critical examination of various traditional tests used in the investigation of female infertility was undertaken, particularly the postcoital test (after a fairly recent act of intercourse, syringe aspirations were made from the cervical canal to assess the quality of the sperm surviving)[4] and tubal insufflation (the patency of the fallopian tubes was checked by passing carbon dioxide or a radio-opaque dye along them). Oestrogen-driven research was extended to assessing women with carcinoma of the breast before and after oophorectomy.[5] This was funded by a grant from the British Empire Cancer Campaign.

At this time, most pregnancy testing was being done using animals, such as the rabbit, the rat or the frog. Such biological tests indicated the large amount of oestrogen in the women's urine in early pregnancy. If this urine is injected into the female rat, the higher level of oestrogen would be detected by changes in the rat's ovaries. This could only be seen after killing the animal and opening the abdomen. Similar testing was done with mice and rabbits but it took time to get a result (48–72 hours), was expensive in animals and was none too reliable. The frog test used male frogs (*Bufo bufo*) and urine was again injected. High oestrogen levels were associated with an ejaculation of frog semen. This took a couple of hours only and, after suitable rest, the frog could be used repeatedly. Hence, it was less expensive but keeping frog colonies was difficult and this test was not used at UCH. These were reasonably secure tests but professionals were looking for a better, more reliable and easier way to perform a pregnancy test in the late 1950s. Swyer worked on the biochemical strip test in its early days.

The research of the Unit on oestrogen levels in the urine as a measure of fetal and placental function continued in the 1960s. Oestrogen levels were easier to measure than those of progesterone and was thought then to be of greater diagnostic predictive value.

In 1959, Swyer and his department took part in a pilot trial on three progestrogens as oral contraceptive agents. This was just a couple of years after the pioneer work done in America and Swyer was among the first of the British workers in this field.

The trial of hormones in oral contraception continued in conjunction with that of Dr Margaret Jackson in Exeter. Now the Council for the Investigation for Social Control took an interest and helped with funding of the first clinical trials on humans using progesterone to prevent ovulation. Although they worked, the doses of progesterones needed were high and made women sick. Oestrogens were added and so the dosage of progesterones could be reduced. The usage of this combined pill was expanded in the early 1960s and much work was done from Swyer's laboratory monitoring this.[6] The basic interest in progesterones continued in the laboratory and clinical studies were run on the synthetic progesteronal compounds, including the assessment of their clinical efficacy and the effects of phases of the menstrual cycle on the endometrium.

In 1961, research supported by the International Planned Parenthood Federation started with low-temperature preservation of human spermatozoa. This was the beginning of the now widely used sperm banks, in which donated sperm was stored in ampoules in liquid nitrogen. These can be used up to ten years later to impregnate a woman. The infertility work was expanded also on the female side to examine the action of the new drug clomiphene, an ovulation stimulator. This non-hormonal drug could be given at the appropriate phase of the menstrual cycle to stimulate the ovary to release several oocytes instead of the usual one or two. Thus the chance of sperm

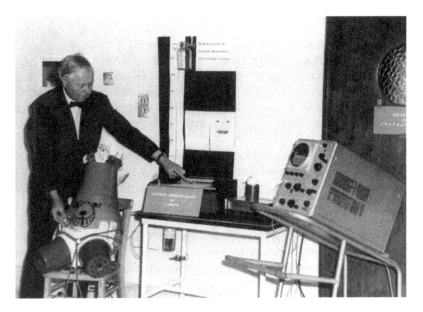

Norman Smyth demonstrating his external uterine pressure gauge at UCH (1960)

fertilising one oocyte was greatly enhanced, but the risks of twin or triplet pregnancies from multiple impregnations had to be accepted.

Swyer was one of Nixon's major collaborators in research. He brought the subject of endocrinology from folklore into science and led UCH under Nixon to be a centre of research in this area. He lived on after Nixon and only retired in 1978.

Biophysics

In an entirely different field of scientific research was Norman Smyth. With his brother, he had been a director of a firm of medical instrument makers (CNS Cambridge). In the Second World War, Smyth had been seconded to the Royal Navy. He worked on radar and received an award from the Royal Inventions Tribunal on the advances he produced. After the War, the brothers decided that one of them ought to have a medical qualification to further their firm's activities. The author worked on the same laboratory bench as Smyth in the Physiology Laboratories at UCL after this in 1948 and remembers him telling how, "We tossed a coin and I lost, so I had to go into medicine".[7]

He went to New College Oxford and then to UCH, qualifying in the early 1950s. He joined the Surgical Unit of UCH where he helped develop experimental machines to measure blood flow in patients undergoing cardiac surgery. He transferred to the Obstetric Unit in 1952 and did research in relation to fetal heart rate activity with a grant from the Nuffield Research Foundation. Norman Smyth made major contributions into fetal electrocardiography, working out better ways to pick up the electrical output of the fetal heart,[8] which is about twenty times less than that of the mother's heart. The latter signals have to be blocked or they would swamp the fetal signal and Smyth tried hard to resolve this problem. It was eventually solved but by workers in Los Angeles and Frankfurt.

Smyth devised a manometer to record external waves of increased intrauterine pressure and this led to the electrical strain gauge ring tocograph.[9] Using two of these, the activity of different parts of the uterus were measurable and the effect of various drugs on them could be assessed. It used to be thought that the cervix dilated passively in labour like a hole in the toe of a stocking being pulled steadily up on a leg. Instead, Smyth showed that the cervix had an activity independent of the upper uterus and that this activity could be influenced by drugs. Arising from this, the combination of fetal heart rate monitoring and uterine contraction measurement was the start of fetal monitoring in labour, which still goes on in labour rooms around the developed world.

At UCH, Smyth tried to develop a wireless transmitting fetal monitoring unit at the nursing station, with input from each labouring mother on different wavelengths, so that they could be walking around the unit or sitting in a room some yards away.[10] Such work was heavily dependent upon clinical assistance with testing the monitors by active obstetricians. Smyth was a shy man and despite Nixon's encouragement, the clinicians often seemed too busy to give him their time. At a later date, Smyth was largely unsuccessful in his pioneering efforts to develop routine clinical cardiotocography in the hospital. His ideas were sound but, lacking clinical clout, he was too dependent upon others to provide the cases and continuity of care he needed. The clinical assistants felt they had far too little uncommitted time available to them to do research.[11] Smyth withdrew into his laboratory and was considered in his later days "a grumpy electronic engineer". This the author considers an unfair judgement – he was reserved but blossomed when taken seriously and by those with a genuine interest in his work. Smyth is recorded as making many sensible suggestions at the Committee for the Co-ordination of Research. These often led to others' projects being improved and showing a significant result.

Research on the external stimulation of the intrauterine fetus led Smyth to shine bright lights through the mother's abdominal wall and, later, to play musical notes with a wireless transmitter. Many women who have been pregnant know of their unborn child's increased activity when loud music is played close to them. There are even those who would claim a differential response to classical music from jazz or popular tunes. Smyth tried to simplify that by using a pure note from a tuning fork (middle C: 512 beats per minute) which he used to place on various maternal bony parts around the abdomen, such as the iliac crest or the pubic bones, to stimulate the fetus by direct vibration and then amplify and record changes in fetal response. The size of response to this stimulus was thought to be a rough guide to the fetal nervous system state but correlations were not very precise.

In 1952, Smyth, at the behest of Professor Nixon, performed research on preliminary ventilation in the newborn. He used a hot-wire amniometer along the lines of Ian Donald's machine that had been developed at the Hammersmith Hospital. He also mirrored Donald's work a few years later in a more widely spread use of biophysics. In 1955, Smyth obtained a grant from the Paul Fund of the Royal Society to further develop what they called an "ultrasonic microscope or telescope", to explore the body with low-intensity ultrasound vibrations "and to make visible the internal structures at a given depth on a television screen". By this time, Ian Donald was already working in Glasgow on obstetric ultrasound but Smyth was among the early people in this country to help turn it into a practical measure. Now, in the next century, nearly every pregnant woman in the United Kingdom has at least one ultrasound to measure fetal size and to look for structural abnormalities in the unborn child and it has since been used widely in general medicine and surgery.

Dynamic studies on measuring head-to-cervix pressures led Smyth to work on medical induction of labour with oxytocic infusions. He took a large part in the research on the efficacy of synthetic oxytocin (Syntocin®). He found this drug to be just as effective as natural oxytocin and without any side effects. The natural product came from the pituitary gland at the base of the brain of the human. These were removed at post mortem and stored for differential extraction in batches. The product suffered from the disadvantage that, at the extraction stage of the natural product, other biologically active constituents passed into the therapeutic process. These caused side effects in about 1% of women but the laboratory-made drug was pure.[12]

The laboratory became a centre for visitors and requests came in from all over the world for workers to join Smyth, as this was one of the few biophysical laboratories devoted to obstetrics. He was in demand from colleagues in France and Germany who were doing similar work and was invited to go to the States permanently to direct a programme of research with Louis Hellman at New York State University. This he turned down. He did, however, travel much in Europe. Once, on a British Council visit to Greece, the wires got crossed and he was billed as a great clinical surgeon rather than a clinical scientist. His hosts produced a woman with a difficult pelvis who was at term. A caesarean section was required. Smyth had seen this performed as a frequent visitor to the operating theatre but never had done one. Nothing daunted, he operated and delivered the baby successfully. There was a corner of Greece after that which believed for many years that in Britain the operation was best done by a vertical incision of both the abdominal wall and the uterus.

In 1958, the support of the Nuffield Foundation for Norman Smyth came to an end. The School Council considered that because of the very fine work being done, they would support Smyth for a while longer to finish off some projects but at the end of September that year he took a joint appointment between the Obstetric and Surgical Units.

Much later, in 1964, Nixon was establishing the Childbirth Research Centre and Smyth returned to its staff full time. He was studying posture in labour, funded by an MRC grant, and working on various aspects of the haemodynamics of labour. The Haines' decompression suit had been introduced to Britain from South Africa. It was supposed to suck up the mother's anterior abdominal wall by external negative pressure, powered by a domestic vacuum cleaner. This, Haines hypothesised, would allow the fetus to line up better with the mother's pelvic brim and so pass down the birth canal more readily with less effort and much less pain. The equipment was assessed and found wanting. Smyth returned to his first love, refining electrical physiological measuring equipment to monitor fetal heart rate measurement and intrauterine pressures; he was still working in the department when Nixon died. Professor Denys Fairweather kept Smyth's tenure going and found university funds for the post. Later they supported Smyth's retirement from the hospital, and the UCH authorities supported his retraining to work in general practice, so as to improve his rather hazy pension provision to look after his wife.

Stimulated by Nixon, who gave moral support when the clinicians seemed to have been ganging up on him, Norman Smyth made an enormous contribution to the biophysics of obstetrics. Having been trained as an engineer and then as a doctor, his emphasis was obviously on the engineering side, which was important. After all, he had a whole hospital full of obstetricians who could have helped him. Some of these felt that Smyth might have consulted them more and in return the clinical staff could have been encouraged to use the fetal monitoring equipment more on the labour ward. Nixon stimulated Smyth's work, giving publicity to his research and helping him with support. Smyth himself was in the forefront of most biophysical work in obstetrics and left the subject much more scientifically orientated than he found it. He was made an honorary consultant in 1965.

Biochemistry

Dennis Hawkins was another of those rare clinical doctors who had sufficient scientific bent and wished to use his science in the clinical field. After second MB, when most students were pressing on to the clinical wards, Dennis Hawkins stayed behind at University College to complete a BSc in physiology and then another two years on top of that for a PhD in pharmacology. He then returned to his clinical studies at UCH and, while he was still a student in obstetrics, he was sent for by Nixon, who had spotted the fact that he had a scientist in the class: "Twenty-four hours later I was in Nixon's office being quizzed about my interests. I expressed a wish to do something on prostaglandins. Nixon found me a laboratory on the top floor, obtained material and equipment for an isolated organ bath, a recorder (invented and made originally by Norman Smyth), a supply of guinea pigs for isolated organ preparations and a supply of specimens from the Fertility clinic".[13]

Hawkins worked in the laboratory every evening when not on call, making standard preparations of prostaglandin and assaying it and attempting (unsuccessfully) to purify the active principal. Hawkins presented his work at the Thomas Lewis Society of the Medical School, a prestigious student society that was particularly concerned with scientific research. However, the rather stuffy chairman of the Society said at the end, "Yes, very interesting, but not quite the thing is it, old man?".[13] It would have been a put down for most young research workers but not for Dennis. Hawkins recalled that, "One day in the mid-1950s Nixon took me down to a lecture at the Royal College of Obstetricians and Gynaecologists, which was then still at 57 Queen Anne Street. He introduced me to one or two people before the lecture as one of his research assistants. A little later, I was in a small group when one said, "Here comes young Will".[13] Nixon must have been over fifty at the time and Hawkins was much taken aback. It made him realise the antiquity of those at the head of the profession.

In 1955, still before Hawkins qualified in medicine, Nixon wanted some research done on the changes in tissue electrolytes in labour, particularly those of the myometrium. He found funds for the laboratory and got Hawkins a technician.[14] This started the work on the electrolytes of the myometrium in labour, which was later expanded to their levels in breast milk. After house jobs, Hawkins applied himself to research on recurrent miscarriage, then called habitual abortion, when a woman has had three consecutive miscarriages with none of her pregnancies going to term. Hawkins and Nixon used to give these women folic acid and B vitamins prophylactically from the time of the first missed period and rest them in hospital for six to ten weeks. This led to many successful live births of large babies.

Hawkins went to Harvard for a year and then to Hammersmith as a research registrar but returned to UCH Obstetric Unit in 1962, staying for three years until he went to Boston as Professor. Much of this later time was taken up teaching and doing the clinical load but he managed to get some further work on uterine activity in relation to isoxsuprine in an attempt to suppress contractions. Some years after Nixon's death, Hawkins returned from Boston and went to Hammersmith, working with Bill McGregor and Professor McClure Browne. He stayed at the Royal Postgraduate Medical School as a consultant and reader in obstetrics.

Haemodynamics

Another major research worker in the department for most of Nixon's reign was Helen Payling-Wright, who was married to George Payling-Wright, the physiologist at UCL. She had been recruited by Nixon to work as a part-time research assistant. Her major interest was in venous blood flow during pregnancy and the blood's clotting properties after delivery or operations.[16] She worked on the factors that led to venous thrombosis using radioactive sodium (Na_{24}) in conjunction with SB Osbourne, the hospital physicist. This localised the site of the reduced blood flow or actual block. Dr Payling-Wright was one of the pioneers in the use of radioisotopes in obstetrics. In those days up to 25 microcuries per pregnancy was thought to be safe. Now we know that there is no safe dose of radioactive materials. She was using Na_{24} to measure venous flow and to determine the sites of clots in the legs. This research was extended to try to isolate sites of high blood flow, such as the placental bed, as this would have a higher collection of blood. Knowledge of the site of the placental bed could be useful, particularly when the placenta might be implanted low down in the uterus, becoming a hazard if vaginal birth were to be attempted (placenta praevia)[17]. Another use to which Payling-Wright put her radioactive isotopes was the rate of absorption by subcutaneous and intramuscular injected solutions. This had important practical implications.

The effect of high- and low-fat diets on blood clotting and the use of anticoagulants also came within Payling Wright's remit[18] and she made valuable contributions in the prevention of deep-vein thrombosis and pulmonary embolism, a major killer after obstetric and gynaecological procedures. Placental site localisation work was abandoned at UCH but taken up in other places. Until the establishment of ultrasound in the antenatal period it was a major method of detecting placenta praevia. Research started with Norman Morris on the quantitative flow of blood into the placental bed and its reduction in pre-eclampsia.[17] The isotope methods were extended to measure cardiac output. As well as her work on the venous blood flow and anticoagulation which was so valuable, Helen Payling-Wright was one of the pioneers for using radioisotopes to measure blood flow to the placental bed and other organs.[19]

Clinical research

As well as these full-time workers, all the clinical members of the department were expected to perform research. A few projects foundered, most others ended in publications but all cannot be recorded in a short volume like this. However, one major piece of seminal research performed by assistants has stood the test of time. John Martin, with Jack Dumoulin, tried to quantify the value of giving prophylactic ergometrine to all women just after delivery of a baby in an effort to prevent postpartum haemorrhage. They compared the blood loss and management of the third stage of labour in 100 primagravidae with normal deliveries who had 0.5 mg ergometrine, given intramuscularly at the crowning of the head, with another 100 women who did not. They were able to show considerable reduction of blood loss with prophylactic ergometrine although there was some increase in the rates of retained placenta, which may have been due to this. However, while bleeding could kill, retention of the placenta did not. This research was repeated with larger numbers and the technique was adopted, thus changing the practice of childbirth worldwide. It has saved many women's lives since.[20]

Research on analgesia and anaesthesia in pregnancy was performed by Shila Ransôm. She tested new equipment such as the portable trilene inhalers and took an active research interest in antenatal education of mothers. The effects of various doses of pethidine, given for maternal analgesia in labour, on the baby's respiratory capacity after birth were investigated. In Nixon's last years in charge of the unit, he encouraged Dr Ransôm to perform a limited trial of continuous epidural analgesia in labour. This went on after his death but UCH was one of the early units to use this technique.

Work was published on breast milk production and breastfeeding by Mavis Gunther. While Norman Morris was chief assistant, he was involved in several projects with other workers but principally he expanded his important work in the psychological associations in gynaecology and obstetrics with outcomes, starting with relaxation in labour.

Before she was first assistant, Pamela Bacon did work on the third stage of labour and delivery of the placenta. She undertook a detailed study on women whose placentas had been delivered by controlled cord traction and she showed this to be associated with minimal blood loss. This was a major contribution to the abandonment in the Western world of the Credé method of placental delivery by forcible uterine compression.[21]

While Denis Bonham's major contribution to research at UCH was the Perinatal Mortality Survey, he kept his clinical research going right up to the time he left for New Zealand. With Dr Maria Grossmann, Bonham started the radiological study of pelvic organs particularly in the cases of polycystic ovary syndrome with gynaecography.[23] This became an established technique at UCH until it was replaced by ultrasonography and diagnostic laparoscopy.

Bonham also devised a system whereby the Schiller iodine test for cellular overactivity in the cervix around the external os could be measured easily. He started testing all expectant mothers coming to the antenatal clinics at 16 and

36 weeks and again after delivery. If the test was positive (that is, a lack of iodine staining) a biopsy was taken looking for malignant or premalignant changes. What Bonham was doing with the pregnant population attending the antenatal clinics of UCH was not really screening. It was an opportunistic testing of a selected group of young pregnant women who were having a vaginal examination for another reason. Screening involved testing a total asymptomatic population of women in the age group more commonly involved in cervical malignancy and premalignancy (40 to 65 years of age). This started the interest in the state of the cervix in pregnancy and Bonham went on to repeat this work, with cervical smears leading to the routine testing of all pregnant women in UK for precancer of the cervix.

With the help of a British Empire Cancer Campaign grant, Bonham started to examine the enzyme levels in the vaginal fluid, comparing them with cervical smears to produce a simple biochemical screening test for cervical cancer.[24] This work came to the attention of Dr Max Wilson at the Department of Health, who found funds for an autoanalyser and the salaries of two technicians to work with Bonham at UCH. This provoked much interest among the gynaecological oncologists at the time. Double testing, comparing this biochemical test with conventional cervical cytology, confirmed the value of enzyme testing. In 4000 tests there was only one false negative but 154 false positive tests.[24] The British Empire Cancer Campaign provided funds for two more technicians but it was at this point that Bonham left for New Zealand. At the same time, the gynaecological cytology service stopped when Dr E. Waters, the histocytologist, retired and was not replaced at that time.

Much other research was done by different workers at UCH. Not all experiments were successful in producing useful results. Dumoulin recalled one such in the early 1950s that had unpleasant side effects and had to be stopped. Before Bradford Hill and Doll's work showing the detrimental effects of cigarette smoking, a large number of women smoked during pregnancy, using "the little red eye of comfort".[25] to relax them from the stresses of the nine-month odyssey. Nixon, thinking that nicotine might help relax uterine muscle also dispatched Dumoulin to the nearby Carreras cigarette factory in Camden Town to negotiate for a batch of cigarettes, unidentified outside but made up with either high or low nicotine levels. Thus, he planned a blind controlled trial with neither the researcher nor the woman knowing the type of cigarette smoked so he could check the effects of various concentrations of nicotine on uterine contractions with the strain-gauge tocograph. Nixon had forgotten, however, another property of cigarette-smoking. For some it is very nauseous and the degree of sickness was also loosely related to the nicotine levels. Soon women urged to smoke three to five cigarettes in early labour were coughing and spluttering and being sick. The study had to be abandoned before any results were obtained.[26]

Other researchers had happier results and Nixon made sure that these were published, forging the final link in a research chain. Having the idea, performing the research, working out the results, then writing it up is no use unless the work is actually published so that all can read it and learn lessons from it. This was where Nixon was so helpful to his staff in directing papers through the right channels to prestigious journals who published them. The record of UCH in obstetrical and gynaecological research over these twenty years was phenomenal.

The Director

Nixon himself took part in much research, although this was obviously limited as the years went by and his talents in other fields were in demand. The researchers had the original ideas but in all cases Nixon had monitored their progress and helped them put papers together. So quite rightly he was considered one of the original research workers from the very time of his onset at UCH. In 1948, he is recorded as doing early work on uterine contractions. Before Smyth joined the Unit and devised his guard-ring tocograph, Nixon used a small tocograph brought over by Professor Lorand from Budapest. Nixon had much faith in this equipment for measuring uterine contractions and so initiating changes in management of labour. The ideas came to the attention of the UCH Magazine for 1948 (volume 23, page 26).

"When a primipara
Loses grip
And her pains
Wains,
If atony from fear
Is near,
Don't curse her
For inertia.
Professor N-x-n
Will fix a
Lorand's tokometre
To defeat her."

Nixon cooperated with Ambrose Rogers of the Mathematics Department of UCL in measuring and recording the weight gain in pregnancy, correlating it with fetal weight. Together with Dr Cecil Williams, they found the mother's starting pregnancy weight to be a better predictor of birth weight than weight gain in pregnancy. Will Nixon realised the value of proper statistical data evaluation in all research and used UCL facilities frequently.

Professor Otto Schild at UCL had synthesised an analogue of oxytocin and he turned to Nixon for clinical trials. He started investigating the action of natural and man-made oxytocin and this is reported with others over several publications. Because of this work and the effort that Nixon put into it, Syntocin® (the laboratory-made drug) replaced the natural product, as has been discussed earlier. This was a major shift in emphasis and Nixon deserves the credit for having persuaded the firm who made it (Sandoz) to give a quantity of the drug to the hospital in order to assess its value. He was irritated, however, when he published the definitive paper a little later on to find that the company had also donated large supplies to other hospitals so that other units were publishing at the same time.[27] This in no way diminished Nixon's work.[12]

Nixon became an early proponent of the metric system in medicine. Until now, drugs and remedies had been prescribed and measured in ounces and minims, drachms and scruples. These measures were obscure, often going back to Biblical days. They bore no logical relationship to each other and only made calculations much harder. They were also open to misinterpretation when written in prescriptions, particularly when added to doctors' well-known poor handwriting and spelling. The metric decimal system was on base ten and had a logical sequence. The original problem was the placing of the decimal point: 0.1 mg is a very different dose from 1.0 mg. In 1949, the Clinical Records Sub-Committee of the Obstetric Hospital had pointed out "the pernicious system of weighing the newborn in grammes but recording their weights in pounds and ounces". This was probably to help the mothers but already Nixon was starting his metrication campaign.[28] It was most successful in the prescribing field where, fortunately, he was backed up by the senior pharmacist at UCH, Thomas Whittet. They led a campaign for the wider use of the metric system in the United Kingdom.[29] This was helped when Whittet became chief pharmacist to the Ministry of Health a few years later and he could use his influence nationally. The first impetus, though, was from Will Nixon.

Nuffield research team

From the mid 1950s, when the Nuffield research team had been established with Norman Smyth and Messrs Farrow and Bainbridge, much of Nixon's direction and participation in research was done through that team. Its publications bore the shared names of the workers. At first, this work was mainly on continuation of recording and measuring uterine contractions or their paucity in uterine inertia. This was followed by research on the induction of labour, the measurement of fetal heart rate activity in fetal distress and neonatal respiration. An oxytocic sensitivity test was elaborated to predict the imminence of labour and indicate the likelihood of induction working.

Unfortunately, in 1958 the support of the Nuffield Foundation ended and the unit had to disband. The research did not stop. Nixon in collaboration with Dennis Hawkins continued a long-term study of uterine electrolytes and the influence of oestrogen and progesterone on their concentrations. In addition, the effect of pathological conditions such as pre-eclampsia on them could be easily measured.

The Childbirth Research Centre

In early 1961, a meeting of a group called the Co-ordination of Research Sub-Committee was called by Nixon with colleagues from Departments of Clinical Physiology, Chemical Physiology, Anatomy and Human Metabolism. Professor Amoroso, Professor Huggett and Alec Bourne were also present. The group decided to initiate a coordinated study into placental function, to assess the risk of intrauterine death from placental insufficiency, and seeking the results of therapy. This was an important advance in the field of obstetric research and led to the establishment of the Newborn Physiological and Pharmacological Research Unit. Financial help came from the Nuffield Foundation and the National Birthday Trust Fund; the laboratories on the top floor of the Obstetrical Hospital were converted into a dedicated unit for this. The National Birthday Trust launched a National Child Welfare Appeal for funds for the Unit and Nixon allocated members of his team specifically to it. However, in 1961, the researchers themselves spent much of their time fundraising as well. Night after night, Nixon would be speaking to groups and charities seeking for funds for his Childbirth Research Centre. All this was on top of being an active teacher and busy clinician and taking his share of emergency cases at night. Some think this contributed to his first heart attack that year.

The name was changed to The Childbirth Research Centre with extra money from the Nuffield Foundation and the Variety Club. A memorandum on articles of association was prepared for the former Board of Trade so that the Centre could be registered as a charity and a National Appeal to raise funds was planned. Unfortunately, this was at the same time as a National Appeal was to be made by the Royal College of Obstetricians and Gynaecologists for funds. Sir John Peel was treasurer of the RCOG then and saw the clash of interests.[30] He was a friend of Nixon and he went, with a small group including Professor Hugh McLaren from Birmingham and Lord Brain, the past president of the Royal College of Physicians, to ask Nixon to postpone his appeal for a couple of years. They pointed out that ,in practice, an appeal from an independent national institution like the RCOG would probably have a greater draw than one for research facilities at one of London's dozen medical schools. Nixon saw this point and agreed.[31]

The Mental Health Research Fund sponsored research into testing of response to stimulus by Norman Smyth. The Medical Research Council supported work in studying posture in labour, The Association in Aid of Crippled Children provided support and the work considered under individual research workers in this chapter related to fetal health was subsumed into the Unit's work. The Nuffield Foundation, the Variety Club of Great Britain and the National Birthday Trust increased their funding and reports began to flow from the Unit about research done there. The volume of research was increasing when Nixon had his last coronary and died in 1966. A Board of Management was set up with Lord Brain as chairman and including Sir Arthur Porrit (past president of the Royal College of Surgeons) and Sir John Peel (then treasurer and a future president of RCOG). About ten notables, such as Sir Wilfred Sheldon the paediatrician, were incorporated. Sir Dougal Baird joined when Lord Brain died, while a very productive businessman, Jim Slater, became chairman. He raised funds actively, making the Research Centre an attractive unit.[31]

In April 1975, the name of this limited company was changed to Birthright by the fundraisers and in June of that year the work of the charity was registered under the auspices of the Royal College of Obstetricians and Gynaecologists as Birthright, later to become WellBeing. It had its own council, with thirteen RCOG members and ten elected by the Council of Birthright. Nixon's successors, Professor Denys Fairweather of UCH and Sir John Peel of the RCOG, were the catalysts of this but the then president of RCOG had not been very keen to start a research centre at the College and so events lay fallow for a few more years. When Stanley Clayton became President, financial negotiations were reactivated by him and George Pinker, now treasurer of RCOG. The Childbirth Research Centre came to the Royal College. Jim Slater took the chair of Birthright Council and its financial executive committee at the time of its transfer to RCOG until he had to retire after financial misfortune in the City. The Princess of Wales became the Principle Patron and Vivienne Parry became the principal fundraiser.[31] In their different ways both were highly successful. This body has since then become WellBeing and is the active charity of the Royal College, distributing over £1,000,000 a year in research grants. All this was started by Nixon's ideas and energies.

The Perinatal Mortality Survey

Possibly the most far-reaching piece of research that Nixon pioneered was the National Perinatal Mortality Survey. While others did a lot of the footwork in this Survey and its analysis, it was Nixon who conceived the idea, ran with it and at all times supervised it in detail, setting up, running, analysis and writing up, always encouraging the workers when the task seemed all uphill. He chose two excellent men to run it: Dr Neville Butler, the paediatrician who had been on the staff of the Obstetric Unit at UCH, and Dennis Bonham, his obstetric assistant there. Albert Claireaux was to be in charge of the pathology. It was Nixon who pervaded the whole study and saw that it worked.

In early 1954, Nixon had the idea of arranging a field enquiry on the relative risks of hospital and home confinement. He and Neville Butler designed a pilot questionnaire and took it to the UCH Committee for the Co-ordination of Research on 8th June 1954. While the general idea was accepted, a large number of suggestions were made in detail if "statistically reliable results were to be obtained" (Professor Penrose). Towards the end of that year Nixon invited representatives of obstetrics and paediatrics and the Ministry of Health, together with the Medical Research Council and statisticians and epidemiologists, to a meeting. It was immediately realised that an enquiry would be very much bigger than was first thought. The National Birthday Trust was approached to see if they were prepared to set up a group to study this problem. Lady Rhys Williams, the chairman and driving force of the National Birthday Trust, saw it as an opportunity to help women and to further the National Birthday Trust's image in the eyes of the public. She arranged that a small grant should be given. A pre-pilot survey was to be done in Norwich to see if such a survey was a feasible way to gather evidence of Nixon's hypothesis.

Richard Law, then one of Nixon's staff who had been a registrar at the Norfolk and Norwich Hospital, remembers that a group of them, including Neville Butler and Will Nixon, drove up to Norwich in Nixon's Ford Consul to enlist support for the pilot study to be done there. After an interview with the senior consultant (and gaining his support) lunch became imminent. The consultant invited Nixon to the hospital dining room but relegated the rest to a café down the road. Nixon would not have this – they were a group and would not be separated. Will said they would all go elsewhere. Law, having worked in the area, was sought for advice. He chose well and so a magnificent lunch, paid for by Will Nixon, was had at the Castle Hotel, after which Law drove the rest back while they slept off their meal.[32]

The National Birthday Trust Committee grew. With Dame Josephine Barnes, an ex-UCH staff member, as Chairman, representatives from all the appropriate medical bodies were appointed and a massive committee was set up to run the survey. Through all these difficult days of manoeuvring Nixon pressed on with "a degree of missionary zeal and drive which was so much part of the survey" and it was this that got the study going.[33] The emphasis shifted from an enquiry into the home-versus-hospital problem to a total study of perinatal mortality in the whole country. This was due to the influence of several epidemiologists, such as Dr Alice Stewart who was then working in Oxford. In fact, the final reports of the analysis never settled the point about the relative risks of hospital and home deliveries; the issue had been lost in the complexities of the survey.

At that time there was a shortage of obstetric hospital beds. About two-thirds of women were delivering in hospital and the other third at home. Members of the House of Commons were asking questions about women being compelled to have their babies at home against their will because of the shortage of beds. It was this political pressure that drove the Ministry of Health into supporting this survey. Lady Rhys Williams made use of her contacts with the Macmillan family (by this time Harold Macmillan was Chancellor of the Exchequer and his son, Maurice, was a Conservative Member of Parliament. Harold Macmillan's wife was a noted political hostess). Meanwhile, events overtook the organisation of the survey. The Cranbrook Committee recommended a 70% hospital delivery rate: 30% short of the RCOG's wish for a total hospitalisation of childbirth. Nixon was very disappointed and at a press conference said, "The Cranbrook Report must not be perpetuated". He attacked the members of the Committee saying, "The next generation will point to them and say "You guilty men".

Meanwhile, Butler and Bonham had been designing and planning the questionnaire of the Perinatal Mortality Survey and had started pilot studies. The final version was very much a clinical document to be filled in by each midwife who supervised a delivery, with some of the questions directed to the mother. A certain amount of antagonism arose between those who were drafting the survey questionnaire and the Committee that was supposed to be in charge of it. Sir George Godber, a wise political doctor, was Deputy Chief Medical Officer at the Ministry of Health. He put his weight behind the survey, realising that it had some advantage to be seen to be coming from some outside source other than the Ministry of Health. Others at the Ministry were not so supportive and it was probably the intervention of Professor Dougal Baird that gave the survey an air of great respectability. Nixon later said that, "Protected by this Aberdonian canopy we felt as secure and viable as the fetus during the mid-trimester of pregnancy".

The obstetrician Dougald Baird was a man Nixon admired enormously. He ran the unit at Aberdeen and, by organising local antenatal clinics under his domain, effectively ran obstetrics for that part of northern Scotland. His team included Angus Thompson, the epidemiologist, WZ Billiewitz, the statistician, Frank Hytten (physiologist) and Raymond Illsley (sociologist). Baird showed by statistical research that the social class of the woman was a major associated variable in the survival of their babies – the lower the social class, with its poor nutritional record, the worse the outcome. Nixon decided to spend a couple of days with him, airing views on what was later to be the National Perinatal Survey. Nixon took Elliot Philipp to Aberdeen with him as he, too, was knowledgeable in this field and was on the scientific committee of the National Birthday Trust. They spent the weekend picking Dougald Baird's brains and discussing embryonic ideas. That weekend started the germination of the survey in the minds of Nixon and Elliot Philipp, which came to fruition at the end of the decade.[34]

However, the Aberdeen caucus was a hard group and the epidemiologist at the Medical Research Council Obstetrical Medical Research Unit in Aberdeen, Dr Angus Thompson, was keen to have full control over all the analysis. A new classification for perinatal deaths was devised to supplement the existing one, which had been pathology-based, telling how the baby died and not why. The new categorisation recorded maternal factors and was able to consider the aetiology of the demise of the fetus as well as the pathological findings. This debate had not been resolved when the survey was actually performed and it was some months later that Angus Thompson wrote to Butler insisting that Aberdeen be given the "Complete responsibility for the whole task of analysing mortality rates…. Long experience suggests that this aim is best ensured by scientific freedom and full responsibility of reproduction being granted to one person: in this case Baird".[33]

Meanwhile, the survey had been performed and data from virtually every birth in England, Wales and Scotland (but not Northern Ireland) during the week 3rd to 9th March 1958 were collected, with a 98% response rate. In addition, in order to consider sufficient perinatal deaths to justify comparisons, all stillbirths and first-week neonatal deaths for the months of

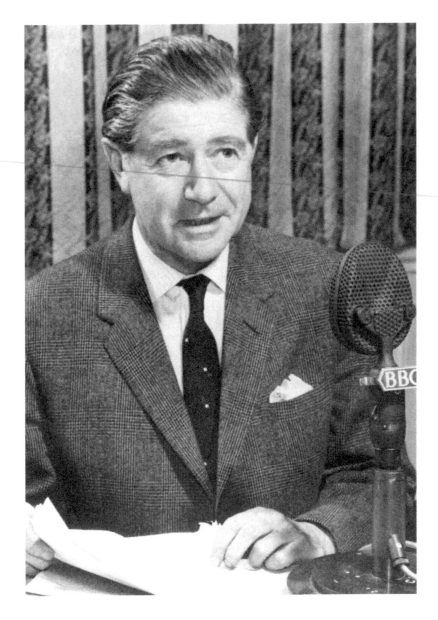

WCW Nixon broadcasting on BBC with the results of the 1958 Perinatal
Mortality Survery (1962)

March, April and May of that year were also included. Thus, 17,205 births in a week were assessed and 666 deaths in three months. The perinatal mortality aspects of this study involved an enormous amount of work on the part of Albert Clareaux, who performed or supervised the autopsies on the babies at perinatal mortality centres throughout the country.

Regional Hospital Boards had distributed questionnaires in advance and the completed forms were checked by midwifery superintendents or supervisors and then by the Medical Officer of Health of the county or county borough area in which the births or deaths had taken place. Often a deficiency could be rectified and missing data were sought. The forms were returned eventually to the National Birthday Trust (despite a postal strike) and eventually some 25,000 completed questionnaires were available for analysis.

No permission had been asked of the mothers for this study to take place, as it was not thought necessary in 1958. There were no ethics committees then and it is probable that neither the mothers nor the midwives understood the concept of informed consent. It was taken for granted that the medical information could be used. The forms were made anonymous by obliterating the mother's name and the mass of data was then checked, coded and transferred to forty-two-column punch cards for all births (this was before the days of computers) by the Government Social Survey staff at the Central Office of Information and also staff at the National Coal Board. Butler and Bonham worked hard on the data, usually after they had finished their clinical duties in the day. Bonham, his wife and his father, also laboured long hours in the night and at weekends on these raw data, producing tables that could be used for analysis. Bonham remembers also how Neville Butler would come to his house in the evening after a clinical day and work through until breakfast.

Harvey Goldstein, a statistician with the National Child Development Study, joined the survey team and introduced multivariate analysis. This shows the association of each factor in turn, independent of the others, washing out a large number of variables so that the important ones can be identified. Several other bodies, some funded by the Ministry of Health, were used to analyse the data. A small editorial committee had been set up. Bonham remembers how Neville Butler was never satisfied and how he was always redrafting.[35] Chapters had to be plucked from him as each was written. They were put on an aeroplane to Edinburgh for the publishers (E & S Livingstone) to prepare proofs. The costs of the freight were borne by the airline: British European Airways.

The first report, *Perinatal Mortality* (published in 1963)[36] was a straightforward account of all the data. Key findings are given in Table 1. At a prepublication press conference held in late 1962, Nixon went into overdrive about the findings, appealing for a crash programme for care of mothers and babies and forecasting a national collapse of the maternity service if the Ministry of Health did not take action: "If we had fifty deaths a week from air crashes something would be done. Yet there are fifty babies a week dying from preventable asphyxia alone". He demanded accelerated recruitment of midwives, improving their status, more maternity beds, early discharge for maternity patients and annexes to hospitals where they could stay if they required antenatal inpatient care. *The Times* quoted Professor Nixon: "The days of removing an appendix on the kitchen table have gone, yet we are perpetuating the same thing in our maternity services".[37] The *Daily Telegraph* referred to the 50 babies born dead or dying within seven days of birth each week in the study. They associated this with the fact that a doctor was present at only one in four deliveries and Nixon again was quoted: "Mothers and babies being needlessly slaughtered. Deliveries were in kitchen table conditions."[38]

Neville Butler tried to cool the press conference by using some solid data about pre-eclampsia and anaemia, and Professor McClure Browne pleaded for more research, but it was to Nixon's words that the press listened and they splashed them over the newspapers the following day. General practitioners (and the British Medical Association) took the report of the whole study as a grave attack on the right of GPs to care for women at home and Nixon's appearance on a wireless interview the following day did little to ease the apparent rift between family practitioners and hospital doctors. Nixon was quoted in the *Daily Mirror*: "You cannot foretell with any woman that something in what looks to be the most normal birth, will not go wrong. All mothers should have their babies in hospital".[39]

The founder and organiser of the Association for Improvement of Maternity Services (AIMS) wrote that a home atmosphere should be made in the hospitals and that nobody seemed to be in overall charge at the Ministry of Health, which was run by committees. At that time, AIMS was not pressing for homebirths.[38]

The final report came out in 1963 and a second volume with a fuller discussion of the results came out later, after Will Nixon's death. *Perinatal Problems* (1969)[40] was written by a team of doctors who ranged rather wider than those who collected the data and the tone is perhaps more measured. The urging for hospital deliveries only was reduced and much reasoned argument was given but the shortage of hospital beds was emphasised.

One of the major good results of the 1958 Survey was the acceptance by the professionals of obstetrics and midwifery of a shorter stay in hospital after delivery. Until this time, fourteen days in hospital after a normal delivery was conventional. After the Kitchen Table Press Conference, the National Birthday Trust Maternity Service Committee suggested reducing this stay to eight to ten days to release beds for inpatient antenatal care. The Committee used the wartime experiences to back its opinion that fourteen days in bed after childbirth was unnecessary. Further, Theobald, in Bradford, for years had been sending 40% of his mother's home at two days with no harmful results and so providing more beds for antenatal women who needed to come into hospital. This was another major contribution that William Nixon's survey made to national midwifery care.

The two volumes, *Perinatal Mortality* and *Perinatal Problems*, are the monuments to an enormous amount of industry by the midwives and mothers in the country who filled in the forms and the workers at UCH, the Ministry of Health and to Aberdeen MRC Epidemiology Unit who rallied to Nixon, its generator. He may have been emotional in his presentation, and of course the press loved this, but the work done led to a re-examination of the maternity services and much improvement in the provision. It was "Nixon's last baby".[30] It is of interest that when Roma Chamberlain and the author compiled the second National Birthday Trust Survey[41] we used almost the same format as Nixon, Butler and Bonham had used twelve years before and so a comparison could be made with the earlier data.

Nixon benefited from the breadth of his thinking about research. He was able to help others to formulate and carry out their work, encouraging them to produce reports and then to publicise their research, as he went around the world talking about them. "You will readily understand how stimulating it was to work in such a powerhouse, all generating from the advanced ideas held by Will Nixon."[42]

Nixon used to liken work at UCH to a tripod whose three legs represented clinical work, research and teaching; the failure of any one leg caused the tripod to fall. John Martin, once having been exposed to the "tripod talk" by Will Nixon, said, "As far as I could make out, all three of my legs had collapsed simultaneously, leaving me frequently sprawling on the floor".[32]

Nixon was able to do his own research and stimulate that of others. This led to many changes nationally and then worldwide. Obstetrics in the twenty-first century owes much to the researches coming from Will Nixon's unit fifty years before.

Table 1. Principal findings of the 1958 Perinatal Mortality Report[36] (prepared by Eva Alberman, an epidemiologist and one of the authors of the second Report, from this survey and published with permission)

MOTHERS' ATTRIBUTES INCREASING THE RISK OF PERINATAL DEATH

Biological:
- Maternal height (lower height, increased risk)
- First or fifth or later born child
- Maternal age (very young or over thirty-four years of age)
- Adverse obstetric history
- Maternal hypertension in pregnancy.

Social or behavioural:
- Father of baby in unskilled occupation or absent (their partners tended to be short and to have more babies at the extreme reproductive ages)
- Smoking in pregnancy.

A mother who was disadvantaged on all these counts had an average risk of perinatal loss over eight times that of a mother who had none of these risks.

BABIES AT HIGHEST RISK OF PERINATAL DEATH

- Babies with congenital anomalies.
- Babies born considerably before their expected date.
- Babies of low birth weight (more often born to mothers at social disadvantage).

PATHOLOGICAL CAUSES

- Lack of oxygen or trauma during labour was thought to account for one-third of the deaths.
- Death before labour and congenital malformations each accounted for another fifth.
- Immaturity, incompatibility between mother's and baby's blood group, and pneumonia together accounted for another 15%.

ADVERSE MEDICAL CARE FACTORS

- The high emergency transfer rate to hospital of mothers of first babies booked for home delivery.
- More than half the mothers, particularly those at high risk, had not received prenatal care until after the fourth month of pregnancy.
- About one-third had had no haemoglobin measurement in pregnancy.
- One in six did not have regular blood pressure measurements.

CHAPTER EIGHT

Teaching at UCH (1946–1966)

I have spread my dreams under your feet;
Tread softly because you tread on my dreams.

He Wishes for the Cloths of Heaven (1899)
WB Yeats

The term 'doctor' comes from the old French *doctour*, which itself is derived from *docere*, the Latin: to teach. For centuries, the art and craft of medicine had been transmitted in an apprentice fashion from senior doctor to junior medical student and so it became the accepted style that doctors taught their juniors. Until the early nineteenth century there were only three universities in England (Oxford, Cambridge and Durham) and they did not bother much with medicine as an academic subject. Then, in a flood in the nineteenth century, many more universities were established, chairs were created in various major disciplines and the teaching of medicine to the undergraduates tended to move under their influence. A university tradition entered medical education, which was then forced into a pattern of lectures and practical classes equivalent in the minds of university administrators to laboratory sessions. Medicine did not fit perfectly as a university subject but only in the last twenty years has it escaped from this mould and now is becoming once more a separate discipline.

After qualifying, the medical teaching of junior doctors is not continued at university level in the UK but left in the hands of the various Royal Colleges. They supervised the training and testing of young doctors on their way through to senior positions and at first there was more emphasis on the assessment than the teaching. Doctors climbing ladders in medicine, surgery and their subspecialties were expected to sit examinations of the Royal College in their own subject. At first there were only two such higher hurdles: the Fellowship of the Royal College of Surgeons or the Membership of the Royal College of Physicians (and their Scottish equivalents). Now there are 115 higher medical diplomas in the UK alone and equal numbers in USA and the Western world.[1] There is a third group of people involved in medical teaching – the patients. In the case of obstetrics, these are the usually well women having babies with their partners. In gynaecology, they are women needing gynaecological treatments. The instruction of all the three groups at University College Hospital was planned and carried out under the aegis of William Nixon, the senior teacher for twenty years. In addition, he and many members of his staff were in great demand to teach at other centres in Britain and around the world.

Undergraduate teaching

As a teacher of students William Nixon was much liked. He had a restless, enquiring mind and his teaching could never be described as routine. He tried to remember the names of all the students who came before him so that he could address them more personally. His ward rounds, tutorials and meetings were always interspersed with contributions from the students.

As well as the clinical teaching, Nixon entered into extramural activities. One particular enthusiasm of his was rugby football, having played himself at St. Mary's Hospital. Often, when the Hospital Cup was being contended in the Spring term, a notice would appear on the UCH Obstetric Department students' notice board, "Professor Nixon will meet **all** his students on the touchline at Richmond at 2 p.m. this afternoon".[2] The author well remembers an occasion when he had to "rescue" Professor Nixon from the hostile hordes who arrived from another medical school. Will Nixon, in his enthusiasm, had led a group of UCH students ostensibly to watch the game but actually to commit mayhem on the students of the rival school. On this occasion, Nixon had made a charge towards the opponents but they outflanked us with soot and flour bombs being propelled with great vigour. The author managed to get Nixon down behind a motorcar with a few fellow students acting as bodyguard to save him from the worst indignities of the white and black missiles.

When teaching undergraduates, Nixon proceeded in a scientific fashion, so that students were made aware of both the traditional medicine and of the latest advances in the science of obstetrics, many of these from his own unit. Beyond this scientific manner, however, his manner of caring for women came through. He always "sat at the bedside adjacent to the patient while doing his bedside teaching, rather than standing and glowering over the clinical victim".[3] So the women were brought into the teaching session. Will Nixon was kind, passionate, helpful and humane. He was a very emotional person; this was near the surface most of the time and perhaps it was what appealed to most of the students who were mostly exposed to rather drier, academic professors. A few of the younger students thought that William Nixon was too emotional in his teaching but this was his strength, as it enabled him to show that he understood the needs of his patients and could transmit this to the students.

For example, he was ahead of his time in patient-centred care. If an episiotomy had to be performed without local anaesthesia (a rare need), he would respond with "How would you feel if the web between your thumb and index finger was cut without anaesthetic?".[3]

His crusades to bring major improvements to the care of pregnant women and reduction of perinatal mortality pervaded his teaching and students remember this side of him most. He encouraged the staff of his parallel departments, such as those of psychiatry, pathology, family planning and endocrinology, to teach the students and was always glad when they took an interest in teaching. Nixon accepted that most students would spend their careers in general practice and so he tried to cater for their needs. Local general practitioners who were skilled in GP obstetrics ran special teaching twice a year.

He was always prepared to listen to students and within the limits of the university education system he would tailor his teaching to what he had heard. He expected the same degree of devotion to his subject to be taken by the students and only rarely was he disappointed. The students who passed through UCH in Nixon's day all came away with a greater knowledge of and interest in obstetrics and gynaecology than those from other medical schools. More people went into the subject and became consultant obstetricians because of the influence of Nixon on their student lives than from any other professor in London in those years. Nixon knew how to flavour a teaching session with humour and anecdote; the stories he told were nearly all based on his personal experience in this country, Hong Kong and Istanbul. They were told with wry humour and often Will would make himself the butt of the joke. He never played down the woman's position as a patient. Occasionally he would tease the students in a gentle way.

Not long after he arrived in UCH, Will Nixon found that the formal systematic lectures and laboratory-style sessions laid down by the university system were not the best way to teach a medical subject. He therefore managed to get the Medical School Council to agree to abandon these, replacing them with an introductory week of structured lectures at the beginning of the six months, which students then devoted to the subject. Nixon referred to this as "laying out the vocabulary and the syntax of obstetrics and gynaecology". After that, for the next few months all teaching was done at the bedside, in clinics or in the operating theatres.

There were regular seminars from 5 p.m. to 6 p.m. on a variety of subjects: perinatal deaths, near-misses (those who had narrowly avoided death) and those who had undergone caesarean sections. As time went by he evolved a system of personal tutors so that a member of the academic staff would be responsible for half-a-dozen students. Again, before the final MBBS Nixon organised a series of pre-examination intensive seminars, with questioning going back and forth in order to accustom the candidate to the interrogation processes. The last ward round before the students took the final examination usually ended with Nixon warning, "Don't forget that when you qualify, the first thing you must do is go straight to the Medical Defence Union with your five pounds [the then subscription] in your pocket".[2]

There were not enough clinical cases at UCH to teach all students practical obstetrics and so, reluctantly, Will Nixon had to negotiate with other hospitals to get his students taught clinical aspects properly. This system evolved so that for one of the two months spent resident in a hospital doing day and night obstetrics, the student would leave UCH to be taught in another hospital where Nixon had trusted friends. In the London region these included Hackney, Maida Vale and the Whittington Hospitals and out of London, Nottingham (before the days of the medical school at that city), Norfolk and Norwich, Bedford and Plymouth.[4] These students would all have a month in the peripheral hospital, with teaching from the medical and midwifery staff there, under the personal care of a consultant who had been a UCH man or woman in their time. In return for their trouble, Nixon would make such consultants honorary lecturers in his department, a small honour but a greatly appreciated one.

Special rounds and seminars were organised. Richard Law, who had moved from UCH to the Whittington Hospital, used to have a special ward round for senior medical students. Dr Desmond O'Neil, an NHS consultant specialising in gynaecological psychiatric problems, would also hold student discussion groups. Dr Spector formed a clinical pathological discussion group so that pathologists of all seniorities would join with students in discussing cases informal setting. This led to a widening of knowledge and information about perinatal deaths and near deaths, thus helping in the care of the living.

The teaching of gynaecology, particularly that of performing a vaginal examination, has always been a problem for women and for medical students. No woman likes having a vaginal examination and to have to have two, one by the doctor who was being consulted and the second by a novice, was a double burden. Nixon tried to reduce this in several ways. Firstly, he would instruct the students about the sensitivity of this examination and how they could take it in their stride. He insisted that they respected the woman's dignity and used to say that the woman herself was nervous enough and if the examiner was also nervous that doubled the effect on both their adrenaline levels. He made students understand that this was a part of real life and, if it was done properly, sensitively and in an understanding way, this reduced the problems.

After practising on models (which were very different from real bodies as they were made of rubber and canvas), he would introduce the students to the women. The women waited in single cubicles, with a nurse chaperone and, if required, a female friend and, after preliminary discussion, they laid down on the couch. Nixon would then position a half curtain across the couch at the level of the woman's waist, so that she was in privacy at her upper end while the examination proceeded at the lower end of her body. The covering sheet was removed and the woman asked to bend her knees. Nixon would demonstrate any external findings that were relevant, displaying the appropriate areas to the students. He would then gently examine with one or two fingers of the rubber-gloved right hand in the vagina and his left hand flat on the lower abdomen. He would try to feel for the uterus, in health a firm regular organ the size of a pear, which, after a little gentle manipulating could be felt between the two examining hands. If it was enlarged, it was even easier to feel. He would move his examining fingers out into either side of the cervix to palpate each ovary in turn (Will Nixon used to teach the students that if they could not feel anything there, the ovaries were probably normal, as anything enlarging the ovary would make it palpable). The student was next invited to ask the woman if he or she might examine and to proceed to follow Will Nixon's example. In this way many students learned how to perform a vaginal examination without much hurt to the woman concerned. For the sake of their future patients medical students have to learn their techniques for pelvic examination and this seemed the most humane way of doing it.

Professor Nixon was a much sought-after student examiner. He would always take part himself in all his own hospital's examinations, something not every senior doctor would do, and he also took part as a visiting examiner in most of the other twelve medical schools of London. In this capacity he also enjoyed examining in Cambridge and for the Royal College of Obstetricians and Gynaecologists in their Membership examination, as well as overseas universities. He was a very fair examiner; he would ask a straightforward question of the student and then listen courteously to the answer. If he thought a student was going off the rails, he would occasionally move in with a verbal nudge and if the student were astute enough they would take the hint and change the line of the answer they were giving. Many students were helped by this and learned their lessons, for an examination is a time of high adrenaline levels and learning for life is often best done at these times. Examiners hunted in pairs and, if Nixon thought his co-examiner was hectoring the student, he would intervene and lower the tone, taking off the heat. Many students were grateful to him for his careful shadowing of his co-examiners.

As Director of the Unit, Nixon was keen on midwives teaching his students. Under the direction of the formidable Sister Billings of the labour ward, he ensured that trained midwives taught the students the elements of midwifery. At one stage he stopped the training of pupil midwives at UCH in order to strengthen his undergraduate medical student training and saw that only trained staff midwives were employed.

The author was taught by Will Nixon. In 1953 at the finals of the MBBS examination I passed medicine and surgery but failed in obstetrics. This was a sadness, as Nixon had me in his office the next morning at 8 a.m. to explain myself. I would have to spend, he said, six months doing obstetrics and gynaecology only and take that part of the examination as a re-sit later in the year. He added, "You will shadow me for the next six months. Where I go, you will go – excepting to the lavatory". Such was the influence this man had on me that at the end of this short apprenticeship I abandoned ideas of other medical specialist careers and went into obstetrics. This gave me a satisfying, useful and happy life that can be directly attributed to the early influence of William Nixon.

Postgraduate education

The doctors who worked at UCH were there not just for helping in the treatment of patients but for training and learning their profession. The junior ones, senior house officers and junior registrars, mostly had their sights fixed on the MRCOG examination, which was taken two or three years after starting obstetric postgraduate training. Those who did this from UCH were nearly all successful; Will Nixon saw to it that they had proper tuition and training in examination techniques. Before the twice-yearly MRCOG examination, a special set of Saturday-morning seminars were run at UCH, mostly by Nixon himself. John Blair, who later became a senior officer in the RAMC and a Reader in the History of Medicine at St. Andrews University, remembers travelling up with another officer from his National Service Military Training base at Cookham each Saturday for this special coaching for the Membership.[5] Nixon always turned up for these sessions and mostly taught the class himself for two hours, laying down principles and encouraging the potential members to think on their feet and derive one logical thought from another.

Once they had passed their Membership examination, Nixon saw to it that these potential specialists were properly trained in the skills and crafts of obstetrics and gynaecology. There were meetings with other professionals such as pathologists and general physicians each week. Pathology meetings took place regularly with Dr Spector examining any deaths that had occurred among babies. All were persuaded by Nixon to display their wares to his department and to a wider field of other doctors who came to UCH for these occasions. The Holme Lectures were continued by William Nixon and these were special occasions at UCH for distinguished associates in reproductive science from other centres to show details of their work in a sympathetic and logical way.

The clinical work of obstetrics and gynaecology went on, mostly performed on the NHS side by the registrars and senior registrars and the lecturers and assistants from the Obstetric Academic Unit. There was much less division between these two sides of medicine than in many teaching hospitals, due to the way that Nixon cooperated with and expected the cooperation of his colleagues in the National Health Service. He took his full share of training of both echelons of doctors. Will Nixon's grand ward rounds were crowded with his academic staff, other obstetric and gynaecological staff members and by visitors to London. On these rounds Nixon shone. He listened carefully to the histories and accounts of the patients' progress given by the medical student, asked one or two pithy questions and then often would launch into an account of some occasion when he had met a similar condition before.

He also used his wit, usually with great tact. On one occasion, a young female doctor had presented to Nixon a case of a married woman who had had a hysterectomy and developed severe prolapse problems afterwards. She suggested they perform an operation on her to cure this prolapse but which would obliterate the patient's vagina. Nixon queried this with a raise of the bushy eyebrows but the young doctor said, "She doesn't need a vagina if she has had a hysterectomy and can't have a baby". Nixon then examined the neophyte from under his beetle brows and said, "I think you had better come to my office after the round and we will have a little talk".[6]

He was innovative in many treatments. As well as the work he did on oxytocics for stimulating the uterus in labour and or damping it down afterwards (see Chapter Seven), Nixon took great interest in the problems of pelvic inflammatory disease. Women with this condition had often been suffering for years with recurrent low-grade infections and, in consequence, adhesions had been laid down between the pelvic organs and other abdominal structures. He used to use tetracycline (in association with a mix of vitamins to stop gastric

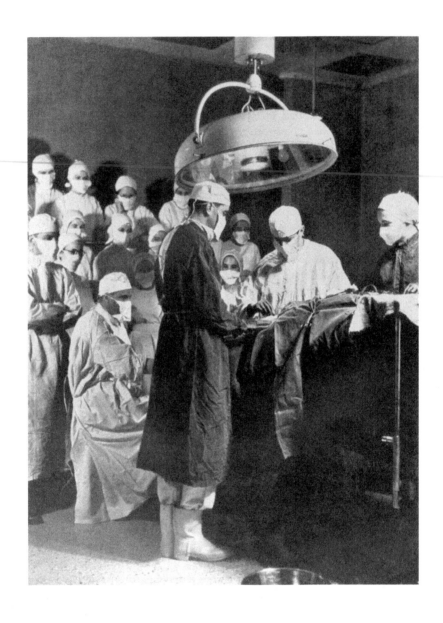

WCW Nixon (in white) operating at UCH (1953)

irritation) and made women rest in bed. Analgesics and short-wave diathermy were added to this regimen and his trainees well remember this. One of them quoted him years later as saying, "There is no quicker way than a hysterectomy to turn a woman with chronic pelvic inflammatory disease into a chronic pelvic woman". He was not obsessed with gynaecological causes for everything. Another of his dictums was, "The commonest cause of backache in women is trouble in the back, not the pelvis".[6]

Having dealt with many varieties of major pathology in Hong Kong and Istanbul, he was well suited to operating on difficult cases. The opinions of his contemporaries about his surgery vary but most of them thought he was very good, particularly at teaching the principles and practice of gynaecological surgery to his junior doctors. He taught surgery by example and precept, always making every opportunity to ensure that his assistant was learning; this applied even to emergency operations in the middle of the night. Once Nixon had established the patient's state was safe and stabilised, he would deal with the surgical problem concerned, such as an ectopic pregnancy, in a logical and clear way so that the assistant could see exactly what was going on. He was against speeding for speed's sake and used to refer to it as "smash-and-grab surgery". Speed came with experience and Nixon would ensure that each step of the operation was done calmly before moving on to the next.

The assistants were expected to dictate to a recording machine a full note of each major operation immediately after surgery. This applied also to all operative deliveries and Nixon saw to it that there were enough working recording machines in all theatres and delivery suites. As well as the account in the hospital records, each assistant then received a note of each operation on a 6-inch by 4-inch card for his own records. From each pathology specimen sent to the laboratory, a copy of the microscope slide would be sent to the assistants' office to examine using the microscope Nixon installed there and so they would learn the histopathology in connection with the surgery while it was fresh in the mind.

He favoured vaginal surgery at a time when that approach to the pelvis was rather in the doldrums in Britain. He thought that this caused less constitutional upset to the woman than did abdominal surgery, and so he used it for hysterectomies, ovarian cystectomies and sterilisations. He realised that such a vaginal approach did not need relaxation of the abdominal muscles (essential for modern abdominal surgery) and so less skilled anaesthesia was required. Having worked in such circumstances, Nixon realised the disadvantages when anaesthesia was not good. He knew his pupils were going to travel widely from the centre of excellence at UCH to other hospitals in Britain and overseas, where anaesthesia might be of a lower quality. Nixon insisted that his assistants always had two helpers at vaginal surgery, to hold and manoeuvre the sidewall vaginal retractors. This would, he said, allow the surgeon to have his hands free and also get a better vision of the area in which he was operating. Once, one of his assistants performed major vaginal surgery with only one helper. Bleeding followed and a haematoma developed; the patient developed a fistula in the bladder after a week or so. The repair of the fistula was carried out by Nixon some weeks later. Drawing the assistant to one side he said, "We will remember to have two helpers for vaginal hysterectomy in future, won't we?" but he never referred to the incident again.

At abdominal surgery, Will Nixon used to teach his staff always to use a Pfannenstiel transverse incision in the lower abdomen, as he claimed it was not only an anti-hernia shutter approach (as the originator intended) but also it ran parallel with peripheral nerves and so did not cut any of them. The scar was very popular with patients in the 1950s onwards for it ran in a gentle curve inside the bikini area. It was Nixon's wont not to have the woman in a very steep head-down position, which was the conventional mark of most gynaecologists. Victor Bonney, the finest British gynaecologist, taught this as being essential to pelvic surgery in order to empty the lower abdomen of the intestines and thus giving a better view. Nixon contended that packs wrung out in warm saline solution could be used instead to hold off the intestines, so giving a perfect view of the pelvis and removing the problems the anaesthetist used to have with the steep tilt which embarrassed respiration.

Like Victor Bonney, his great hero, Nixon advocated conservation in surgery. He used to remove benign cysts from ovaries, leaving behind the outer ovarian capsule and repairing it by turning it in so preventing the raw tissue edges encouraging adhesions. He used to remove fibroids from the uterus widely (myomectory) rather than perform a hysterectomy, and he expected his staff to follow these examples. In fertility work, Nixon followed the principles of Green-Armytage when performing tubal surgery to restore the patency of the oviducts that carried the fertilised ovum to the uterus. He was not keen on undertaking surgery for malignancy. Quite rightly, he thought that if you were going to do such operations you should be performing them frequently. Hence, Nixon used to concentrate this work under Tim Flew, his NHS colleague and later under Jo Holmes, who was also a very good operator. Any radical vulval surgery for cancer he would send down to the London Hospital, as Alan Brews' team was particularly good at it and they gained more experience in radical vulvectomies as a consequence.

However, Nixon was perfectly capable of performing such surgery and once when Jo Holmes was away for a long interval, a woman appeared with advanced carcinoma of the cervix and an ovarian cyst. This could not await Holmes' return and Nixon arranged to do a Wertheim radical hysterectomy on her. A couple of newly arrived young doctors, thinking that Nixon's surgery might be suboptimal, watched, "… to see what kind of a mess the old boy would make of it". They came out of theatre two hours later crestfallen for they had to accept that Nixon had done a masterful job and they had never seen a Wertheim operation performed so skilfully.

When cervical smears became widely used Nixon thought it would be a good idea to invent an instrument to take a small biopsy of the cervix of those women with a positive smear. It was a simple tool; a metal rod with a grip on the end which would take a small portion of a razor blade. Nixon encouraged his assistants to use this tool. When one cut his finger quite severely, Nixon asked another assistant to try it but to be not so clumsy. The second assistant suffered the same fate. Nixon was not pleased and at the next operating list he said he would use it himself to show how it should be done properly. At this third attempt, Will Nixon cut his own finger quite badly, and so he gave in and discarded the instrument.[6]

It was Nixon's ambition that all his assistants should fly the nest as professors and consultants in other parts of the UK and the world. They would be missionaries of his philosophy and few of them did not so succeed. Several remember that, after a few years of his tutelage, Nixon would start to drop hints to them over tea in the afternoons. Several record being called to his office to be told that a professorship had been arranged for them in some other part of the world. In some cases it was taken with alacrity but for some it did not suit family plans. However, Nixon was determined to spread his disciples wide. The ideas that Nixon inculcated in the minds of his youthful assistants stayed and long after his death the Nixonian way of doing something in obstetrics and gynaecology persisted.

Nixon had himself trained for and had taken successfully the examination for the Fellowship of the Royal College of Surgeons (FRCS) during his time as a resident as St. Mary's Hospital. It was conventional then for all gynaecologists who wished to get on in teaching hospitals in London to have done so and FRCS became the norm. Later Nixon opposed this, saying that the training required for the Membership of the Royal College of Obstetricians and Gynaecologists was sufficient and that the Fellowship was a distraction that was not necessary. Hence, he did not encourage his own staff to put themselves forward for the examination and since then the need for an FRCS in general surgery has been seen to be unnecessary by most gynaecologists.

The women coming for treatment

The third group of people to whose teaching Will Nixon set his mind were the women themselves – those having gynaecological treatments and women coming forward for a safe and happy delivery. In the first group, Nixon was careful that any woman who was going to have an operation had it explained to her fully in the outpatient department by whoever was recommending it. Knowing that sometimes the mind goes blank on these occasions, Will used to insist that when women came into hospital (waiting lists were short in those days), whoever was to perform the operation would ensure personally that the woman had it explained to her a second time before surgery and certainly well before the preoperative drugs were given, as these might confuse her understanding. He would often sit beside the woman with pencil and paper drawing the proposed operation and explaining the point of it. Nixon was most unusual in the 1940s in doing this but many women who were under his care were helped. Now it is the expected procedure.

Women who were going to deliver at UCH were invited to attend antenatal classes. At the Professor's behest, Mrs Helen Herdsmann, the physiotherapist, started educational preparation classes; all were invited to join. Nixon invited the expectant mothers and the fathers to attend classes and the professor spoke to the first class himself. Too often in labour, the father had been left out and everything was done for the mother; all concerned themselves with her pregnancy and her labour; father, perhaps, felt he was less important. Nixon considered it was correct that mothers and fathers should meet him for not only was he Director of the Unit responsible for the classes but he was in charge of all treatments. Subsequent classes were mostly performed by midwives and physiotherapists. Nixon provided the class teachers with birth atlases and model pelvises as visual aids. Such detailed teaching of women having babies was unknown in the 1940s and Will Nixon introduced it to UCH, making sure that women were well informed. It also gave them an opportunity to think about the subject and to express any worries they might have.

After Nixon had settled in as Director of the Obstetric Unit at UCH, he discovered that women admitted antenatally for rest were woken between five and six o'clock every morning. This was so that the night staff could get them sorted out, given their breakfasts and medicines before the day staff came on duty at 8 a.m. Nixon went into battle over the next three or four years and finally won, so that women admitted antenatally were allowed to sleep until 8 a.m. Sadly, the midwives managed to slip the times back over the next two or three years and they were being woken at 6 a.m. again.

The most anxious time for most women in the whole of pregnancy is childbirth itself and so much emphasis of the teaching was placed upon the labour. Nixon used to insist that the women were told certain details, such as the fact that no castor oil was given in the hospital (In the 1940s this was a standard method of clearing the bowels before labour; it was thought to have some stimulating effect on the uterus). He also insisted that women knew there was no danger that their babies would be confused with any other baby from the delivery suite. Each was labelled on the wrist before leaving the labour room and then lived with their mothers afterwards in the lying-in ward, staying all day.

Relaxation instruction was started with special reference to Grantly Dick-Read's ideas. Classes were taken jointly by Dr Shila Ransôm, the anaesthetist and the physiotherapist, who talked openly about pain in labour and how it could be reduced. They also emphasised the need for relaxation and how it would help in the relief of pain particularly in the last part of the first stage of labour. Usually a woman would attend four or five antenatal classes and about 60% of women managed to achieve this. It was felt by the staff of the labour rooms that such instruction was helpful to women and that they had an easier time in labour than those who knew nothing of what was going on. Nixon was one of the first to bring husbands into their wives' deliveries provided both wanted it and, as Nixon himself used to say, "…there was no arm- twisting". Fathers were asked to agree to leave if requested without necessarily thinking anything had gone wrong with his wife or the forthcoming baby. Once, a father fainted, fell to the floor and fractured his jaw so that while his wife returned home in ten days, he had to stay in hospital until six weeks later.

Will Nixon turned UCH from being much more than a highly technical research institute of obstetrics and gynaecology into a centre for teaching of medical students, doctors and women. He was most enthusiastic about it and insisted on no dropping of standards even in the face of staff shortages. If a staff member could not turn up for an instruction session, rather than interrupt the pattern of teaching Nixon would go down to the classes himself at no notice. His warm, friendly attitude towards women helped him in this.

"He was a kindly and compassionate man whose life was devoted to the welfare, happiness and health of women. At the same time, he was under no illusions about the fair sex as it was presented to the gynaecologists of the

1950s."[6] This is the lasting memory that Dennis Hawkins, one of his assistants, has of him fifty years later. It sums up Nixon's desire not only to improve standards by teaching attention to detail and quality in the technique but by also helping the women understand what was going on in childbirth or a gynaecological operation.

CHAPTER NINE

Nixon the Man (1928–1965)

And walk among long dappled grass,
And pluck till time and times are done
The silver apples of the moon
The golden apples of the sun.

The Song of Wandering Aengus (1897)
WB Yeats

William Nixon presented many personalities to many people. He was a complex man but basically a humane one. No one with whom the author has spoken has a bad word to say about him. He was courteous, with elegant manners, and looked after the interests of his women patients, his students, his family and his visitors. He loved his fellow men and women. He had a great love of country and expressed it wherever he went. He was a stimulator of research and he fostered this in the young. Anyone who had an idea could discuss it with him. Nixon was prepared to challenge the establishment and introduce *avant garde* innovations. If he appointed someone, he trusted them and showed them the moral courage of his support. "Will was generous in extreme. He was also a courteous and modest man. He expected a high standard of constructive advice if any criticism was offered and it was not his habit to destroy but to build."[1]

Nixon had a wandering soul; he moved his professional base several times, including long stays in appointments in Hong Kong and Turkey. In these, his love of his fellow men enabled him to take advantage of the best that was going in these places. Even after being appointed Professor at UCH he wandered actively, returning to Malta often and travelling to visit departments in all parts of the Commonwealth and the world – lecturing and advising but at the same time picking up new ideas. In this, he was a great advocate for Britain, which shows in his addresses and lectures outside the country.

He was a social man and loved to meet with people who flocked to his unit in later days. He loved entertaining and sharing the pleasures of the table. He was a member of the Savage Club, where he liked to escape the confines of the

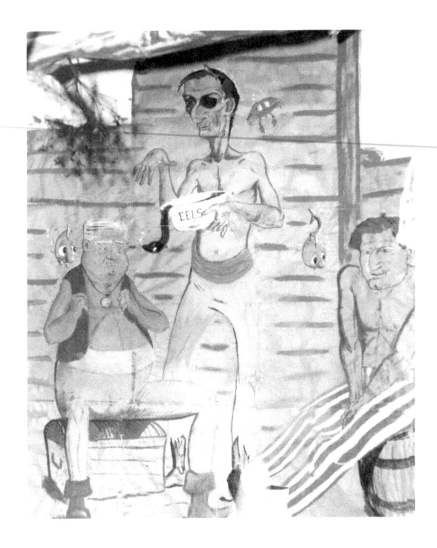

A part of the scenery from the Fallopians Student Review of 1953. WCW Nixon is seated on the left with his two chief assistants. John Martin enjoys his favourite fish, eels, while Jack Dumoulin sits on the right (provided by Professor John Martin of Perth, Western Australia)

medical world; Wendie, his daughter, remembers seeing the Coronation of King George VI from there. The Club was then in an enormous imposing house in the Mall. Nixon would entertain his staff at clubs and restaurants like *L'Escargot* and the *Café Royale*. John Martin remembers one memorable evening when Will Nixon took out a group of senior assistants with Norman Smyth to outline new research proposals requiring the clinicians' cooperation. After an excellent meal with a lot of wine, Norman, who had a weak head for alcohol, said that he had drunk too much to be coherent and would prefer to postpone the discussion. The others in equally cheerful mood all agreed readily and the research component was postponed for a few days.

Nixon did have other bolt-holes nearer home and UCH. After the day's work was done, he would gather some of his staff and visit one of the local pubs, where he would entertain them with anecdotes which were, if not always tactful, invariably amusing and well received.[2] The Copper Kettle in Wigmore Street was a favourite and is still there. He would sometimes slip down Gower Street into Store Street where the famous Italian restaurant, Olivetti's, always welcomed him and his guests for long lunches. Nixon had been of some professional help to the proprietor's family and they never forgot that.[2] Occasionally, he would lead a group down to a real Chinese restaurant in

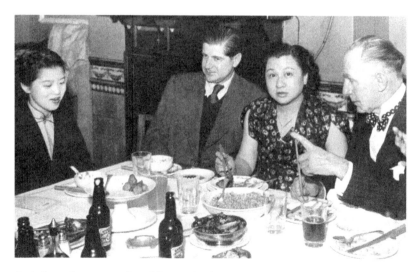

An informal supper at the Old Friends Chinese Restaurant in Whitechapel. WCW Nixon is with two visitors from Hong Kong and Green Armitage of Hammersmith Hospital

Whitechapel. Home entertaining was a little limited, as neither Vennie nor Sidi liked large parties; they were both were much happier with a small number of good friends. Sidi was described by many as a lovely and very attractive woman who became friends with his staff, but after Will's death she retired somewhat and eventually withdrew completely. She lived very frugally, surviving to 2000.

Nixon's extrovert manner encouraged caricatures. Each Christmas, the medical students at UCH held a satirical show called "The Fallopians" in the UCL Theatre. In 1952, many of the sketches parodied the Obstetric Hospital and its staff. The scenery was painted by John Hogben, portraying the seniors in the Obstetric Unit. Jack Dumoulin sits on the left with Nixon on the right with a fish in his ear. Standing is John Martin devouring a bowl of eels, his favourite dish. The author was stage manager of that show and well remembers one verse of a skit about Nixon, to be sung to the tune of *It ain't necessarily so*, from George Gershwin's musical, "Porgy and Bess":

> "I favour the student who cares
> A great deal about his repairs*
> If you don't then soon yer
> Will get dyspareunia**
> And similar trouble downstairs."

Professor Alan Boura, a pharmacologist working at UCH with Nixon, remembers a more permanent illustration:

> It was decided to compare the effects of oxytocin and vasopressin on the uterus of women having their pregnancies terminated for therapeutic reasons so there could be no likelihood of the hormones having adverse effects on the developing fetus. A multi-tubed sterile catheter with six small balloons was introduced under anaesthesia into the uterus. Each balloon was filled with

---

*During their obstetric training, students, after a little instruction, used to suture all tears in the perineum and episiotomies ("repairs") as a matter of course. Some were neater than others but all took time. Now this task is performed by trained midwives.

** Pain accompanying intercourse.

water and connected by water-filled rubber tubing, running across the operating theatre floor to recording pressure manometers on a trolley against the wall. Either oxytocin or vasopressin in small doses was injected into an arm vein of the patient.

My main job besides setting up the apparatus was, gowned, capped and masked, to circulate around the operating theatre persuading people not to lean against the trolley holding the manometers which made them record inaccurately nor to stand on the six rubber tubes running across the floor. If the latter occurred, the tubing compression sent large pressure waves down to the manometers also ruining recordings.

The patient had been anaesthetised, the catheter inserted and its tubes connected to the recording manometers. Professor Nixon thought that the level of anaesthesia was not sufficient and asked the anaesthetist to increase its depth. As more anaesthesia was given, the patient's uterus apparently exhibited a series of violent contractions. Nixon wheeled round from the patient to the watching students and launched into an extremely erudite description of what he thought was the reason why the extra anaesthetic was causing the effect. It was difficult to interrupt his flow for sufficiently long for somebody to gently point out that a junior probationer nurse was standing on the tubing. Nixon gave a terrible glare over his mask at the offender, shook his head, and snorted before turning his attention to the patient. The probationer, in obvious fear and trembling, no doubt wished the floor would open and swallow her up. In those days, one went in terror of giving professors offence.

William Nixon was not allowed to forget his gaffe. It was nearly Christmas and somebody, no doubt full of Christmas good cheer, painted an enormous cartoon with Mercurochrome on the white operating theatre wall. At the end of the table was standing a remarkably good likeness of Nixon, with catheter in hand. A bubble over his head contained the legend, "I can prove anything with this little catheter. Once published, my news will astonish the world". Behind him a particularly voluptuous probationer had a delicate foot poised on the tubing running across the floor.

Mercurochrome is a vivid red dye, used as a skin antiseptic before surgery and it was a long time before the cartoon could be painted over. Meanwhile it was noticeable that Nixon confined himself to discussing each patient's condition, rather than assessment of recordings. Eventually these quite clearly demonstrated that oxytocin was superior to vasopressin for stimulating the uterus to induce labour.

Nixon would proceed from work to one or another of the social venues in his battered Ford car. He was renowned for his volatile driving: "Being driven through Central London by Nixon is an experience not to be forgotten – he made taxi drivers around Trafalgar Square look like amateurs".[3] His daughter remembers well a trip that William Nixon shared with her to Stratford upon Avon and the Warwickshire countryside on a holiday from school at the age of fourteen. As well as the historical castles and the theatrical aspects of Stratford on this trip, Nixon's driving was also an unforgettable memory.[4]

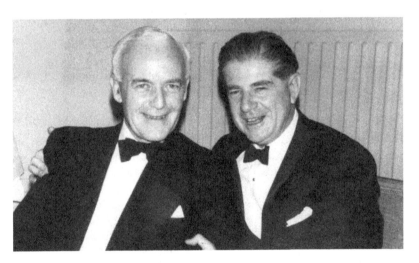

WCW Nixon with George Davidson of Aberdeen at a meeting of the Gynaecological Club in Cardiff

The Professor was a member of the Gynaecological Club, a travelling club in the United Kingdom that obstetricians and gynaecologists were invited to join, not just because of their intellectual standing, but because of their sociability. They would visit centres in this and other countries to watch surgeons operating and having joint scientific meetings, but mostly entertaining each other in the evenings. Will Nixon was always a leader in this entertaining as he had plenty of convivial spirit. He was remembered particularly for his active rendering of a song, the last line of each chorus ending with "… but she couldn't tell Stork from butter". When he died he was greatly missed: "The sorrow will be felt particularly by his fellow members of the happy band of travellers, The Gynaecological Club. Nothing delighted him more than to receive hospitality from gynaecologists abroad and in due course to return that hospitality in Britain. Many have happy memories of parties at the Royal Society of Medicine and the Savage Club and of the fun we and his other guests enjoyed, although basically, Nixon was serious minded".[5] William Nixon went out of his way to look after visitors from overseas both in his hospital and afterwards. He recognised the loneliness of some who were far from home and ill at ease. Nixon was a great ambassador whether he was in Britain or abroad.

Nixon enjoyed his wines and his food. He would mockingly complain, "Oh, those lovely sauces". These sauces contained cholesterol and fats, which may have played a part in his coronary artery occlusion. He lived, however, in an age before we measured those things, when our doctors worry us about cholesterol in food and our future health. Many of these good things are the fats and chemicals that provide the flavour of foods. Nixon knew this and enjoyed them. He made a notable trip to the vineyards of France for a week organised by André Simon. His great friend George Bouchard of *Bouchard Aine* of Beaune, guided him to the best restaurants and vineyards in Burgundy. After his first coronary thrombosis, Nixon was overweight. Much of this had started in Turkey fifteen years before. He was told firmly by Rosenheim to slim. For example, all wines were to be cut from his diet and replaced with two whiskies a day. He was rationed to two eggs a week and became very thin.[6] Like the other medical advice he was given – to ease up his hard professional life – Nixon could not.

In all these years at UCH, Nixon lived in very comfortable areas of London. According to the hospital authorities, he was supposed to live within three miles of the hospital. Before the War and in his early consultancies he had a flat at 64 Harley Street. This was on the sunny side of the road and in a popular block of the street. He used to see a few private patients there, although he did not approve of private practice in principle Nixon took this as part of the job when he was a part-time consultant. He later established a great dislike of what was going on in the Street, particularly for those teaching hospital consultants who left their NHS commitment to their registrars while spending their time in Harley Street in paying practice.

After Hong Kong he came back to Rivermead Court, a large block of elegant Victorian apartments next to Hurlingham Club in Fulham. Long after Will was back from Istanbul, Vennie stayed in South Africa, until 1948. Nixon wanted a divorce but Vennie was reluctant. On her return to the UK they separated.

His future wife, Sidonie, became a naturalised British citizen in December 1946 and changed her name by deed poll to Nixon in January 1953.[7] At that time they were living in Longford Place in St. John's Wood. Will and Sidi were married in September 1955.[7] Vennie moved to Oxford where she died, aged fifty-seven, in 1956. Their daughter, Wendie, went to St. Mary's School, Calne, in Wiltshire. Nixon had taken the trouble to seek out the headmistress, Elizabeth Gibbons, who had run a school in a prisoner-of-war camp in Hong Kong under the Japanese. He was so impressed with this that he considered her an excellent choice to supervise the education of his daughter. In the early 1950s, the Nixons took a flat at the top of 25 Wimpole Street. Like many other properties of that age in that area it had an antique lift that went up to the third floor and then you had to walk up stairs to the top flat. This had many memorabilia of jade and ivory carvings from the Chinese days.

The professional life of William Nixon was crowded with honours. He was an honorary member of obstetric and gynaecological societies in Athens, Belgium, France, Turkey and Uruguay, as well as the Medical Society of China and the Obstetrical Society of Hong Kong. He gave the de Lee (the man to whom Grantley Dick-Read had dedicated *Revelations of Childbirth*) Memorial Lecture at the Chicago Lying-in Hospital and later that decade was the guest speaker at the Association of Obstetrics and Gynecology in California. He was an Honorary MD of the University of Bristol and his external university examinerships show the regard in which his peers held him.

He was made a Commander of the Order of the British Empire (CBE) in 1965, an honour that was richly deserved. His reply to one of the many letters of congratulations received said, "There were many others who should have been selected. I look on it as a sign that obstetrics and gynaecology is becoming recognised as equal to medicine and surgery and other disciplines".[8]

This last was a subject about which he felt strongly. Two days before he died he returned to it in a letter to Norman Morris: "There is still much to be done, as you know, to stake the claims of our subject to be on a par with surgery and medicine … to demote the subject would really be a catastrophe. What is obstetrics other than applied medicine? Is there any other aspect of medicine in the wider sense on which reproductive physiology and pathology must impinge? As I see it this is going to be our next challenge, may you have many years of happy endeavour".[9]

Nixon was a great humanitarian, "His travels were to persuade him of the universality of mankind, which was evident by his welcome of all who visited his clinic, whatever their colour, from all over the world. Few personalities have been so endowed with grace and charm, humour, intellect and genius for friendship. His knowledge of man and the wide range of his reading and interests in arts made his conversation always informed and instructive".[10]

He was a great believer in the fact that it took two people to make a baby and therefore two people should have the baby. He was among the first to encourage husbands into the labour wards for delivery. This was at a time when other professors in London were saying that husbands should be banned for, as Professor John McClure Browne used to say, "They will bring in germs on their boots". Visiting in Nixon's lying-in wards was liberal, especially for fathers. However, it was restricted in the late morning and early afternoon, as the mothers need some rest and peace in a day full of new baby and congratulating friends. Nixon arranged that one of the first to visit the woman after birth would be the hairdresser. When a woman was to be discharged home with her baby after delivery, Nixon would arrange that the couple could go out the night before for a special dinner in a local restaurant. The baby would stay, being looked after in the nursery, while the husband and wife went out. This was very popular with the patients of the unit, of whom there were many, and indeed the practice was used by many of us later in life.

A fine measure of a hospital's consultants can be made by noting who the hospital staff themselves consult for medical care. All the UCH doctors used to try to get their wives booked under the care of Will Nixon, as they knew of his humanity. He delivered Jonathan Miller's family and also took on as NHS patients other people, like Jo Grimond's wife. As a university professor, William Nixon could book no private patients. Many opulent women, British and foreign, booked as NHS patients with Nixon, as all received the same care.

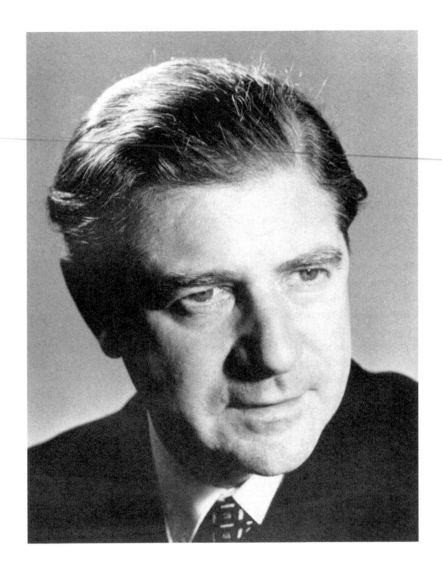

WCW Nixon in 1960

Nixon championed many causes of a humanitarian nature. He was very unhappy at the dropping of the atom bombs that finished the War and was greatly pleased by the introduction of the National Health Service to Britain in 1947 following the Beveridge Report of 1942. He spoke avidly about care of people and how the Health Service had improved that, especially the maternity service. He also felt strongly about termination of pregnancy, saying that women who did not wish to go through with their pregnancies for social as well as medical reasons should be helped with termination. He was named, "the Abortionist of Huntley Street" by his detractors, who mostly worked in Harley Street and "the Illegal Abortionist of Gower Street" by ill- informed protagonists of the Pro-Life Movement. This was not a fair description, as no abortions done at UCH were illegal. He applied the principle that Alec Bourne had catalysed and developed and which the courts had formulated about consultation by two doctors. Nixon was quite strict, always to be aided by a psychiatrist, Keith Soddy at first and Elizabeth Tylden later.

Alec Bourne, Nixon's mentor, friend and confidant had, in 1938, decided to test the law. Until that time, abortion or the attempt to cause an abortion was a crime under the Offences Against the Person Act of 1861. Bourne had been consulted by the parents of a fourteen-year-old girl who had been raped by three soldiers. He decided it was in the best interests of the girl's health that pregnancy should not continue. He informed the Metropolitan Police that he intended to perform a therapeutic abortion and went ahead. After the surgery, he was arrested and appeared at the Old Bailey. After a closely argued case, the Judge, Mr. Justice McNaughton, ruled that, "Doctors may terminate a pregnancy if the risk to the mother's health, physical and mental, is greater than the continuation of the pregnancy". This then became case law (*obiter dictum*) for all judges below the Court of Appeal. Hence, since Nixon always had medical or psychiatric agreement from another doctor and good reasons for termination of pregnancy, the proceedings were not illegal. The Pro- Lifers were ill-informed and incorrect.

Women turned to Nixon because they knew they would get a fair evaluation instead of being turned down flat or asked for a lot of money. He openly supported the movement that led up to the Abortion Act and, although this did not come into force until after his death, he advocated it at meetings in the House of Commons to MPs, discussing both the problems and relative merits. Some at the extremes of religious and ethical thought became his enemies over the Abortion Act but he still supported the principle. Nixon was irritated with the ideas of the Roman Catholic Church on abortion and contraception, possibly arising from his years in a Catholic-dominated country: Malta. He thought they were out of step with the needs of both the developed and the developing worlds.

The same groups also castigated Nixon on being a member of the English Eugenics Society, under the mistaken advice that Eugenics equalled racial cleansing. This also was nonsense; Nixon was a member of that intellectual group which welcomed Dougal Baird, Maynard Keynes and Julian Huxley. The Germans may have given Eugenics a bad name under the Nazis but this distinguished group of social scientists was working towards a better world, not a more restrictive one. They examined all the biological factors that existed and led to the evolution of society. Such unthinking misinformation as the Pro-Lifers put out about Nixon is still given space in this century and, in the author's opinion, does not deserve serious attention.

One fascinating thing about Nixon was that he managed to do things so discreetly and quietly that one did not find out about them until much later. He was involved with the opening of an escape route for Jews from Bulgaria and Romania to Turkey and on to Palestine during the last War. He had hoped to write about this in his memoirs when he retired to Malta.[11]

Another episode which shows Nixon's strong humanitarian views on issues is one that very possibly accelerated his death because of the stress involved, after he already had a coronary thrombosis. One of the doctors who had worked with Mengele in the Nazi death camp at Auschwitz in the Second World War had been involved in sterilisation experiments on both men and women using radiation of the gonads, to find a minimum dose which would stop them from childbearing. This was all part of the Nazi purification-of-the species philosophy. When the War finished, that doctor left Germany, worked in the Far East and then returned to North London. Leon Uris, a noted American writer, had found out about this and had written a veiled account of it in a book entitled *Exodus*, which was first published in 1959. In it, he stated that the experiments had occurred on women and that, "Dr Dehring had performed 17,000 experiments in surgery without anaesthetics". Dehring sued the publishers of the book and Mr Uris for libel and the case appeared in the High Court before Mr. Justice Laughton and a jury in April/May 1964.[12]

Some of the women had been re-examined by Professor Nixon. These women, having been irradiated, later had their ovaries removed under anaesthetic in order to examine the organs microscopically and so assess their capacity to produce eggs. Nixon appeared as a witness for the defence on the grounds that what had been written was true, of public interest and not a libel. He became quite emotional about the injustice of what had happened to the women and the inhumanity of the operations, which he considered had taken place. Giving evidence-in-chief in answer to Lord Gardiner QC, who appeared for the defendants, Nixon outlined the necessary steps required in a pelvic operation to remove the ovaries. He discussed the eight women whom he had examined before the case and it was during questions about the length of the incision that Nixon started to become upset. When asked by Lord Gardiner how the scars of these eight women would compare with those you would expect to find from women operated on in England he replied, "Well, I have practised in England, China, Africa and the Middle East and never in all my surgical life have seen such scars as I saw last week. When I examined the patients there was gross scarring and tissue deficiency".[12]

Events worsened when Gardiner, slightly provocatively, asked if ever a surgeon would be justified in carrying out an operation which he knew was not required for any legitimate medical purpose against the will of the patient. Nixon replied, "It would be completely contrary to my practice and that of my colleagues anywhere in Europe. Since for the last 2,400 years we have subscribed to the Oath of Hippocrates who by example showed the world what responsibility for medical action was and even in the 1940s most of us still subscribed to the Hippocratic Oath, 'I will use treatment to help my patient according to my ability and judgement but never with a view to injury or wrong doing … I will abstain from abusing the bodies of men or women either free or slave'".

In response to the judge, Mr. Justice Laughton, when asking if he had to do such a job under constraint, could he minimise the evil effect, Nixon replied, "I have never found myself in such a situation and I hope I never shall. If I had to perform such a mutilating operation unnecessarily, the crime would remain with me for the rest of my life and I just wonder if I would be able to live up to such a situation". In cross-examination, the subjects of the size of the scar and the speed of the operation were again raised. Nixon stated that at least a four-inch incision was required to give adequate exposure to remove the ovaries, ligate the stumps of the pedicles and cover them over, "All obstetric surgeons would share that view, unless they were so conceited as to boast of their celerity". An incision of two or two-and-a-half- inches was far too small. Surgeons who used such a small incision would be, in the witness's view, incompetent. Finally, cross-questioned on whether the incision would not depend on the nationality of the surgeon doing the operation, Nixon replied, "I would not have thought it had any association to nationality. It is just crude, bad surgery".

This was taken up by the Judge in the summing-up. The jury was out for two hours and they found for the plaintiff. When asked, "What sum do you award against the defendants?" they answered, "One halfpenny". This was really a slap in the face for the plaintiff and implied that the jury thought that Dr Dehring might not have been technically guilty but morally he had offended greatly and damages of one halfpenny (0.5p) were a considerable snub. Further, the plaintiff (Dr Dehring) should pay the costs of the case. Rough justice thus had been done but the emotions raised by this case were many and Nixon's cardiovascular system took a terrible strain from it. His medical advisers felt that the second coronary, which he suffered a little later, had been exacerbated by the court proceedings. They tried unsuccessfully to persuade Nixon to start an easier life.

For all the professional attainments, the research and the teaching that Nixon did perhaps the last word should rest with an unknown colleague, who in an additional note to the anonymous obituary in the Lancet said, "In his care for mother and baby, Nixon would provide a deep compassion: but then nothing but the best was good enough. No one could doubt he was working for his patients".

CHAPTER 10

Last Days

Outworn heart, in a time outworn,
Come clear of the nets of wrong and right;
Laugh, heart, again in the grey twilight,
Sigh, heart, again in the dew of the morn.

Into the Twilight (1923)
WB Yeats

William Nixon was not a well man in his last years; his heart was failing. He had been a powerful athlete in his younger days, a rugby football forward and a great swimmer, both of which tend to lead to heavy body and arm muscles. He was still a good athlete in his adult years: witness his swimming the Bosphorus when he was over forty. However, the years of good living with the rich foods and fine wines were taking their toll. He was overweight and under stress.

Nixon's first heart attack occurred in 1960 when he was in Bath for the weekend. He was taken to the Royal United Hospital from the Francis Hotel in Queen Square where he was staying. He had been under the care of Max Rosenheim (by this time Professor of Medicine at UCH) for hypertension. Max considered it his duty to go down to the West Country to see Nixon. Had the estimation of cholesterol levels and other more modern biochemical criteria been available, these might have strengthened Rosenheim's hand in advising his reluctant patient, but such tests were not yet developed. The treatment used for an acute heart attack in those days was morphia for the pain, oxygen if the patient was cyanosed and strict bed rest with very gradual return to light duties. While the first two may have been given, the third was probably not fully carried out, as Nixon was back at work within a few months. When he returned, he seemed grey and feeble and deteriorating, while on his ward rounds he was withdrawn. He did not visit the labour ward or go to the operating theatre. By this time, the first accounts of Thalidomide causing a peripheral neuropathy (damping down the peripheral nerves in the limbs) were appearing in the medical journals. A cardiologist in Bath had put Nixon on this drug as a sedative not realising these adverse effects. He had thought it was perfectly safe in the male patient but, as well as causing

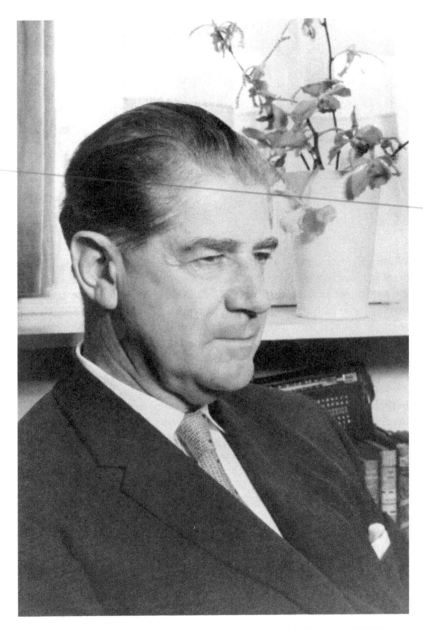

The last portrait of WCW Nixon, taken three months before his death (1965)

abnormalities of the fetus in pregnant women, it also affected the nerves of the body of both sexes and obviously Nixon had developed such a problem. He thought that he was liable to have a stroke and stopped taking the drug. Within a week or two he was back to his former self and shouldered again responsibility for running the Unit and many external commitments.

In 1964, soon after the stormy release of the first results of the National Birthday Trust Perinatal Mortality Survey and the libel case in which he gave evidence, he had another coronary thrombosis, while staying in Brighton. Again, he was put to bed for strict rest but he used to sneak out to the telephone to speak with Mary Alexander, his secretary, who kept him in touch with what was happening at the Obstetric Unit in his absence. She was extremely loyal to him and preserved his secrets.1 He took too little time off duty and it was then that Dennis Hawkins, who was about to take up his appointment of Professor in Boston USA, went down to see him. "He was confined in bed in a single room and seemed pleased to see me. When I told him that I hoped to return to London after four years in Boston, he got quite agitated and told me off. I think he had a vision, in many ways justified, of his assistants going abroad to act as permanent missionaries. Nixon then said, 'London obstetrics is going into a decline from which it will take twenty years to recover'. How right he was." [2]

He returned to work a little shaky but determined to press ahead with his grand idea of the Clinical Research Unit at UCH. By this time, a large part of the operative load had been passed by Nixon to his first assistant, Don Menzies, whose surgical skills he strongly supported. For such a sensitive patient as William Nixon, Professor Rosenheim was perhaps a little tactless when he greeted his colleague's return to London from the second heart attack with, "Don't worry, Will, Don Menzies has looked after the department well since you have been away". [2] Because of his general ill health, Nixon was concerned he might be retired, as he thought that he was the victim of petty jealousy in the upper hierarchy of UCH doctors. Such a premature end of his professional career would not have been his wish, for although he wanted to retire to his beloved Malta in the fullness of time, he did not feel that he was ready yet. He had bought land there but no house was yet built. Nixon was quite concerned that his post at the University College Hospital was insecure and while there were others on the medical staff who did not see eye-to-eye with him, there is no evidence that this actually was so.

On New Year's Eve 1965, Will Nixon invited for interview in his flat, Herbert Brant, a young doctor from New Zealand who had been working in

Hammersmith Hospital. After a long interview, Nixon offered Brant the post of first assistant, as Menzies was returning to Liverpool in the New Year. Herbert Brant and his wife Margaret were planning to return to New Zealand for a short holiday but in February 1966 they received a telephone call to say that Nixon had died and Brant was wanted to take over the Department of Obstetrics and Gynaecology as soon as possible as an interim measure. He was given consultant status and moved into UCH. Here, he was helped with the teaching by Tony Woolf and Ernie Kohorn, the senior lecturers. He appointed Rosemary Utidjian as an extra lecturer.[3]

Nixon's third and fatal heart attack occurred on 9th February 1966 when he was sixty-two years old. There was a committee meeting at the Obstetric Hospital about the method of selection of Nixon's successor. The chairman turned to Nixon and said that he hoped that this was not embarrassing him, Will Nixon rose to his feet and left the room replying, "I only hope I will not be embarrassing you". We do not know whether the beginnings of chest pains were already coming on but he walked to his office in Chenies Mews (100 yards away) and was already suffering his final coronary thrombosis.

Howard Baderman, later a consultant in accident and emergency medicine, was at that time the Resident Medical Officer at UCH, the senior of the resident doctors on the medical side of the hospital and a previous house surgeon of the professor. He remembers Nixon bleeping him to tell him that he had had another coronary. In those days there were no well-trained and practised mobile cardiac arrest teams available and so Baderman ran across from the main hospital to Chenies Mews. Nixon's office was on the first floor and Baderman hurried in only to find that Nixon was dead. His shirt was open and he was slumped over his desk; apparently his pupils were dilated and he was cyanosed. There was nothing that could be done and so Baderman sadly made his goodbyes to his old chief and started to make arrangements for others to collect the body.[4] Tim Flew remembered that the committee meeting had been an acrimonious one and it could easily have been that which precipitated events.[5]

There was a quiet family funeral and Nixon's remains were cremated. A little later on Friday 11th March 1966, a memorial service was held at Marylebone Parish Church.[6] This is one of the large square metropolitan churches on busy Marylebone Road. It was full of obstetricians senior and junior, his patients and all who had worked in medicine with Will Nixon, perhaps notable for the large number of senior registrars from many of the teaching hospitals at the back, the author among them. The list of the great and the good is long. Principal among them were the family of William Nixon, led by his widow.

Lord Amery, the Senior Physician at UCH, and Sir Douglas Logan, Principal of London University, led the official mourners. The President of the Royal College of Obstetricians and Gynaecologists, Sir Hector Maclennan, was in Australia and so the College was represented by Sir Arthur Bell (immediate past president), Sir John Peel (immediate next president), Humphrey Arthure, senior Vice President, and Tom Lewis, Honorary Secretary, with many other past and present members of Council. Sir Arthur Porritt (a St. Mary's man and Honorary Fellow of RCOG) read one of the lessons. He represented the Royal College of Surgeons. Sir Cecil Wakeley was there on behalf of the Imperial Cancer Research Fund, while Lady Micklethwait and Miss Doreen Riddick represented the National Birthday Trust. Lady Medawar attended with Sir Theodore Fox (Family Planning Association) and Sir Arnold Walker from the Central Midwives Board. The Medical School was represented by Dr Arthur Holman, Chairman of the Medical School Council, and Peter Verill, Vice Dean of the Medical School. The Matron of UCH and many members of the medical, midwifery and nursing staff were present, together with a large number of medical students and nursing students. Dr ET Spooner was from the London School of Hygiene and Tropical Medicine and Dr W Thomson represented the journal, *The Practitioner*. Dr DC Bowie came from the British Postgraduate Medical Federation and Thomas Whittet, by now Chief Pharmacist at the Ministry of Health, represented that Ministry. Mrs Rettie represented the International Planned Parenthood Federation and Dr Margaret Suttill the British Council. The Headmaster of Epsom College, Mr. AD McCallum and Dr D Deas, President of the Old Epsom Club, were there. Dr Donald Tear represented the Medical Defence Union while Professor Hugh McLaren came from Birmingham and AM Fisher from Bristol. SA Wood came from the Royal College of Midwives and Miss Hylton-Jones from the Obstetrical Association of Chartered Physiotherapists. She had been once in charge of the obstetrical physiotherapy at UCH.

The clinical load had to go on at the Obstetric Hospital and the staff coped. Professor Bert Brant was hastily appointed to the staff. His interests were in the psychosomatic field and Brant filled in for the late Director until Denys Fairweather from Newcastle arrived as Nixon's successor in the autumn of 1966. He continued with his research into the rhesus factor and perpetuated William Nixon's teaching. Fairweather also looked after the Childbirth Research Unit, ensuring it a good home in the RCOG later.

Now, Nixon's memory is preserved in a ward of the Obstetric Hospital named after him and by his picture in the medical school. He catalysed many people to follow his ideas about obstetrics. Many consultant obstetricians throughout the world carried on with the principles he taught and the practice he showed them. Nixon left his mark on obstetrics, not in a series of publications or the writing of great books, but in his personal capacity as a human being to influence other human beings. It still shows.

APPENDIX 1

The chronology of William Nixon's life

YEAR	PROFESSIONAL ACTIVITIES	DEGREES, HONOURS	OTHER ACTIVITIES	UK AND WORLD EVENTS
1903	Born 22nd November		Malta	Edward VII
1905				
1910				George VI World War I
1915				
	Epsom College		UK	
1920				
	St. Mary's Hospital Medical School	Epsom College School		
			Marriage to Vennie	
1925		LRCP MRCS		General Strike
	House Surgeon, St. Mary's Hospital			
	House Surgeon Great Ormond Street	FRCS		
1930	Resident Medical Officer, Queen Charlotte's Maternity Hospital			
	Registrar, St. Mary's Hospital	MB MD (Gold Medal)		UK financial collapse
	Registrar, Queen Charlotte's Maternity Hospital	MRCOG		
	Outpatient Surgeon, St. Mary's Hospital			
1935	Outpatient Surgeon, Queen Charlotte's Hospital			
	Professor, Hong Kong		Hong Kong	George VI
	Surgeon, Soho Hospital for Women & Consultant, St Mary Abbott's and Paddington Hospitals	FRCS		
				World War II
1940				
			Blair Bell Lecture, RCOG	Bombing raids
	Professor in Turkey			

YEAR	PROFESSIONAL ACTIVITIES	DEGREES, HONOURS	OTHER ACTIVITIES	UK AND WORLD EVENTS
			Istanbul	V1 & V2 raids
1945				
	Professor at University College Hospital		UK	
				National Health Service introduced
1950	World Health Organization Maternity Care Committee		de Lee Lecture, California	
			Marriage to Sidi	
	Council of the Royal College of Obstetricians and Gynaecologists			Elizabeth II
	Ministry of Health Special Advisory Committee on Maternity Care			
1955	Vice President, British Medical Association O/G Section			
	National Birthday Trust Survey		Ceylon	
1960			Coronary thrombosis (1)	
	National Birthday Trust Survey Published		Auschwitz court case	
		CBE	Coronary thrombosis (2)	
1965				
	Died 9th February 1966		Coronary thrombosis (3)	

APPENDIX 2

The publications of William Nixon

Compiled from *Index Medicus* and UCH Obstetric Unit reports

1931 Calcium therapy and the toxaemias of pregnancy.
The Lancet ii:291–2.

Influence of age on labour.
Journal of Obstetrics and Gynaecology of the British Empire 138:821–6.

1934 Menstruation and its relation to disease.
The Practitioner 132:356–65.

1936 Postpartum haemorrhage.
Clinical Medical Journal 50:1829–34.

Lithopaedion.
Journal of Obstetrics and Gynaecology of the British Empire 143:821–6.

1937 Oedema in pregnancy.
Chinese Medicine Journal 52:317–28.

Aids in the diagnosis and treatment of ectopic gestation.
British Medical Journal 2:579–81.

1938 Oedema of pregnancy.
Journal of Obstetrics and Gynaecology of the British Empire 45:48–59.

Prevention and control of puerperal sepsis.
The Practitioner 141:785–8.

With McCance RA.
Diet of the expectant mother – clinical experiences.
Public Health 51:364–6.

1939 Diagnosis and treatment of disproportion.
The Practitioner 142:163–70.

1940   Endometriosis of the bladder.
The Lancet i:405–6.

1941   Diet in pregnancy (Blair Bell Memorial Lecture).
Journal of Obstetrics and Gynaecology of the British Empire 48:614–35.

1942   With Wright MD and Fieller EC.
Vitamin B1 in urine and placenta in toxaemia of pregnancy.
British Medical Journal i:605–7.

1944   Practical application of knowledge of nutrition to pregnancy and
lactation.
British Medical Bulletin ii:100–1.

1946   With Eckstein A.
Congenital malformations.
British Medical Journal i:432–3.

With Laqueur W and Basat M.
Goblk Hemoglen.
Oleusunun Degeri 27:12.

Early recognition of disease: complications of pregnancy.
The Practitioner 157:215–18.

With Newton TH and Theobald G.
Water metabolism in pregnancy.
Proceedings of the Royal Society of Medicine 37:558–68.

1947   Antenatal and postnatal care.
Ceckoslov Gynack 26:445–52.

With Egeli E, Lagueur W and Yahya J.
Icterus in pregnancy.
Journal of Obstetrics and Gynaecology of the British Empire 54:642–52.

Management of delay in labour.
Proceedings of the Royal Society of Medicine 61; 311–16.

1948   Diet in pregnancy.
Journal of the Royal Institution of Public Health 11:27–33.

1949   Advances in midwifery.
The Practitioner 163:274–81.

1951   Uterine action – normal and abnormal (de Lee Lecture).
American Journal of Obstetrics and Gynecology 62:964–84.

1952   With Bill GH.
Abnormal uterine action in labour.
Journal of Obstetrics and Gynaecology of the British Empire 59:617–62.

1953   Antenatal care; advice for expectant mothers.
British Medical Journal i:268–9.

With Whitet TD.
Metric system in medicine and pharmacy.
British Medical Journal i:327–8.

Hormone de Croissance et Grossesse.
Bulletin de la Societe Royale Belgique Gynecologie et Obstetrie 23:293.

Aspects physiologiqest cliniques de l'action uterine.
Bulletin de la Societe Royale Belgique Gynecologie et Obstetrie 23:318.

1954   Psychosomatic preparation for childbirth.
Proceedings of the Royal Society of Medicine 47:385–7.

Venous thrombosis in obstetrics and gynaecology
Ibid Venous thrombosis in obstetrics and gynaecology
Ibid 25:321–33.

Weight control and toxaemia of pregnancy.
Postgraduate Medical Journal 31:266–71.

Dynamics of the uterus and its clinical applications.
Proceedings of the Royal Society of Medicine 48:674–81.

1955   Social factors in obstetrics.
Bulletin de la Societe Royale Belgique Gynecologie et Obstetrie 25:87.

1956   With Bainbridge WN, Schilds HO and Smyth CN.
Synthetic oxytocin.
British Medical Journal i:1133–5.

With Ransôm S.
Physiotherapy and antenatal care.
Physiotherapist 41:239.

Menstrual disorders as psychosomatic manifestations.
The Practitioner 177:589–97.

1957   With Smyth CN.
Physiological and clinical aspects of uterine action.
Journal of Obstetrics and Gynaecology of the British Empire 64:35–46.

With Hawkins DF.
Uterine electrolytes in pregnancy and labour.
The Lancet 272:837–8.

With Pearce JD and Anderson EW.
The psychiatric indications for termination of pregnancy.
Proceedings of the Royal Society of Medicine 50:321–7.

With Hawkins DF.
Blood electrolytes in prolonged labour.
Journal of Obstetrics and Gynaecology of the British Empire 64:641–8.

With Steward HC, Hughes WH and Thomas EG.
Trichomonas vaginalis: clinical trial of a mixture of an antiseptic
with local anaesthetic.
The Lancet 273:1028–30.

1958   With Bainbridge WN and Smyth CN.
The effect of rupture of membranes on length of labour.
Journal of Obstetrics and Gynaecology of the British Empire 65:189–99.

With Smyth CN.
Oxytocin in obstetrics and gynaecology.
Triangle, Sandoz Journal of Medical Sciences 3:239–49.

With Hawkins DF.
The electrolyte composition of the human uterus.
Journal of Obstetrics and Gynaecology of the British Empire 65:895–910.

With Hawkins DF and Whyley GA.
Uterine electrolytes in pre-eclampsia.
Journal of Obstetrics and Gynaecology of the British Empire 65:911–16.

1959 With Smyth CN.
Old and new methods for induction of labour and premature labour.
American Journal of Obstetrics and Gynecology 77:393–405.

With Walker A, Kimble N, Muir CJ and Embrey MP.
Use and abuse of Ergometrine.
Proceedings of the Royal Society of Medicine 52:566–74.

With McIntosh JM, Walker CW and Wood A.
The general practitioner in the maternity services.
The Practitioner 183:79–83.

With McIntosh JM, Walker CW and Wood A.
The general practitioner in the midwifery services.
Proceedings of the Royal Society of Medicine 52:711–20.

1960 Family planning and population pressure in Ceylon.
Family Planning 9:15–18.

1961 With Hawkins DF.
The influence of oestrogen and progesterone on the electrolytes of
the human uterus.
Journal of Obstetrics and Gynaecology of the British Commonwealth 68:62–7.

With McLaren HC, Attwood ME, Bonham DG, Macrae DG,
Hawkins DF and Eton B.
The cervix – intrapartum and postpartum.
Proceedings of the Royal Society of Medicine 54:712–20.

With Bainbridge MN and Smyth CN.
Fetal weight, presentation and progress in labour.
Journal of Obstetrics and Gynaecology of the British Commonwealth
68:738–54.

1962 Dogum trevayiunin oxytocin ile enduksiyonu.
Sigorta Saglik Dergial Turk 15:458.

1963 With McNaughton MC.
Obstetricians please help obstetrical research.
Developmental Medicine and Child Neurology 5:72–4.

1965 The challenge of perinatal mortality.
Medical Digest 3:94.

Books

Nixon WCW and Ransôm S (1951)
Relief of Pain in Childbirth. London: Cossalls.

Nixon WCW and Hickson P (1953)
Guide to Obstetrics in General Practice. London: Staples.

Nixon WCW (1955)
Childbirth. Duckworth Medical Health Series.

Nixon WCW and Chamberlain GVP (1964)
Childbirth (revised edition). London: Penguin Books.

APPENDIX 3

The Staff of the Academic Obstetric Unit, UCH headed by WCW Nixon from 1946 to 1966

(Compiled from UCH reports and partly from contemporary medical directories)

1946

Director (full time)	WCW Nixon
Assistants (part time)	Miss Aileen Dickens
	Miss Josephine Barnes
	Miss Gladys Dodds
Registrar	EWC Buckell

1947

Director (full time)	WCW Nixon
First Assistant	Miss Aileen Dickens
Assistant (part time)	Miss Josephine Barnes
	L Williams
	H Malkin
	Miss Gladys Dodds
	HH Fouracre Barnes
Registrar	IT Fraser

1948

Director (full time)	WCW Nixon
First Assistant (full time)	Miss Aileen Dickins
Assistants (full time)	Miss Sheila Martin
	AB Swarbreck
	JG Dumoulin
Assistants (part time)	Miss Josephine Barnes
	Miss Gladys Dodds

Unit Obstetric Registrars	HH Fouracre Barnes
	IT Fraser
	TB Fitzgerald
Research Anaesthetist	Dr Shila Ransôm
Research Assistants	GIM Swyer
	Dr Helen Payling Wright

1949

Director (full time)	WCW Nixon
Deputy Director	Miss Josephine Barnes
Assistant (full time)	JG Dumoulin
Assistant (part time)	IT Fraser
Registrar	TB Fitzgerald
Research Anaesthetist	Dr Shila Ransôm
Research Assistants	GIM Swyer
	Dr Helen Payling Wright
	HH Fouracre Barnes

1950

Director (full time)	WCW Nixon
Deputy Director (part time)	Miss Josephine Barnes
Assistants (full time)	Miss A Dickens
	JG Dumoulin
	JD Martin
Assistants (part time)	TB Fitzgerald
	AE Ealamond
Research Anaesthetist	Dr Shila Ransôm
Research Assistants	GIM Swyer
	Dr Helen Payling Wright
	HH Fouracre Barnes

1951

Director (full time)	WCW Nixon
Deputy Director (part time)	Miss Josephine Barnes
Assistants (full time)	Miss A Dickens
	JG Dumoulin
	JD Martin
Assistants (part time)	TB Fitzgerald

	AE Ealamond
Research Anaesthetist	Dr Shila Ransôm
Research Assistants	GIM Swyer
	Dr Helen Payling Wright
	HH Fouracre Barnes

1952

Director (full time)	WCW Nixon
Deputy Director (part time)	Miss Josephine Barnes
Consultant Endocrinologist	GM Swyer
Assistants	JG Dumoulin
	H Pells Cocks
	J D Martin
Research Anaesthetist	Dr Shila Ransôm
Research Assistants	Dr Helen Payling Wright
	HH Fouracre Barnes

1953

Director (full time)	WCW Nixon
Deputy Academic Head (part time)	Miss Josephine Barnes
Consultant Endocrinologist	GM Swyer
First Assistants	JG Dumoulin
	NF Morris
Assistants	H Pells Cocks
	JD Martin
	RG Law
Research Anaesthetist	Dr Shila Ransôm
Research Assistants	Dr Helen Payling Wright
	HH Fouracre Barnes
Research Assistant (Endocrinology)	Miss H Braunsberg
Nuffield Research Assistant	C N Smyth

1954

Director (full time)	WCW Nixon
First Assistant	NF Morris
Consultant Endocrinologist (part time)	GM Swyer
Research Anaesthetist	Dr Shila Ransôm
Pathologist	PE Hughesdon

Assistants	Miss Josephine Barnes
	JD Martin
	RG Law
	RT Martin
	J Elstub
Research Assistants	Dr Helen Payling Wright
	HH Fouracre Barnes
Research Assistant (Endocrinology)	Mrs H Braunsberg
Nuffield Research Assistant	C N Smyth
Steroid Chemist	Miss MI Stern

1955

Director (full time)	WCW Nixon
First Assistant (full time)	NF Morris
Consultant Endocrinologist (part time)	GM Swyer
Assistants (full time)	RT Martin
	J Elstub
Research Anaesthetist	Dr Shila Ransôm
Pathologist	PE Hughesdon
Research Assistants	Dr Helen Payling Wright
	HH Fouracre Barnes
	RG Law
Nuffield Research Assistant	CN Smyth
Steroid Chemist	Miss MI Stern

1956

Director (full time)	WCW Nixon
First Assistant (full time)	NF Morris
Consultant Endocrinologist (part time)	GM Swyer
Assistants (full time)	J Elstub
	HE Reiss
Research Anaesthetist	Dr Shila Ransôm
Pathologist	PE Hughesdon
Research Assistants	Dr Helen Payling Wright
	HH Fouracre Barnes
	RG Law
Nuffield Research Assistant	CN Smyth
Steroid Chemist	Miss MI Stern
Endocrine Research Assistant	Miss J East

1957

Director (full time)	WCW Nixon
First Assistant (full time)	NF Morris
	WG MacGregor
Consultant Endocrinologist (part time)	GM Swyer
Assistants (full time)	HE Reiss
	CAB Clemetson
Research Anaesthetist	Dr Shila Ransôm
Pathologist	PE Hughesdon
Research Assistants	Miss Cicely Williams
	Dr Helen Payling Wright
	HH Fouracre Barnes
	RG Law
Nuffield Research Assistant	CN Smyth
Steroid Chemist	Miss MI Stern
Endocrine Research Assistant	Miss J East

1958

Director (full time)	WCW Nixon
First Assistant (full time)	WG MacGregor
Consultant Endocrinologist (part time)	GM Swyer
Assistants (full time)	HE Reiss
	CAB Clemetson
	Miss Pamela M Bacon
Research Anaesthetist	Dr Shila Ransôm
Pathologist	PE Hughesdon
Research Assistants	Miss Cicely Williams
	Dr Helen Payling Wright
	HH Fouracre Barnes
Nuffield Research Assistant	CN Smyth
Steroid Chemist	Miss MI Stern
Endocrine Research Assistant	Miss J East

1959

Director (full time)	WCW Nixon
First Assistant (full time)	WG MacGregor
	JD Martin
Consultant Endocrinologist (part time)	GM Swyer
Assistants (full time)	CAB Clemetson

	Miss Pamela M Bacon
	JR Saunders
Research Anaesthetist	Dr Shila Ransôm
Pathologist	PE Hughesdon
Research Assistants (part time)	Dr Helen Payling Wright
	CN Smyth
Endocrine Research Assistant	Miss J East

1960

Director (full time)	WCW Nixon
First Assistant (full time)	JD Martin
	Miss Pamela M Bacon
Consultant Endocrinologist (part time)	GM Swyer
Assistants (full time)	JR Saunders
	DG Bonham
Research Anaesthetist	Dr Shila Ransôm
Pathologist	PE Hughesdon
Research Assistants (part time)	Dr Helen Payling Wright
	Mrs Ellen Grant
Endocrine Research Assistant	Miss J East

1961

Director (full time)	WCW Nixon
First Assistant (full time)	Miss Pamela M Bacon
	DN Menzies
Consultant Endocrinologist (part time)	GM Swyer
Assistants (full time)	JR Saunders
	DG Bonham
	JF Leeton
Research Anaesthetist	Dr Shila Ransôm
Pathologist	PE Hughesdon
Research Assistants (part time)	Dr Helen Payling Wright
	Mrs Ellen Grant
	Mrs Valerie Little
	Mrs Agnes HS Onions

1962

Director (full time)	WCW Nixon
First Assistant (full time)	DN Menzies
Consultant Endocrinologist (part time)	GM Swyer
Assistants (full time)	JR Saunders
	DG Bonham
	JF Leeton
	DF Hawkins
Research Anaesthetist	Dr Shila Ransôm
Pathologist	PE Hughesdon
Research Fellow	GW Theobald
Research Assistants (part time)	Dr Helen Payling Wright
	Mrs Valerie Little

1963

Director (full time)	WCW Nixon
First Assistant (full time)	DN Menzies
Consultant Endocrinologist (part time)	GM Swyer
Assistants (full time)	JR Saunders
	DG Bonham
	DF Hawkins
	RW Beard
	KA Harrison
Research Anaesthetist	Dr Shila Ransôm
Pathologist	PE Hughesdon
Research Fellow	GW Theobald
Research Assistant (part time)	Mrs Valerie Little

1964

Director (full time)	WCW Nixon
First Assistant (full time)	DN Menzies
Consultant Endocrinologist (part time)	GM Swyer
Assistants (full time)	JR Saunders
	DF Hawkins
	DG Bonham
	AH Labrum
	KA Harrison
Research Anaesthetist	Dr Shila Ransôm
Pathologist	PE Hughesdon

Research Fellow	GW Theobald
Research Assistant (part time)	Mrs Valerie Little

1965

Director (full time)	WCW Nixon
First Assistant (full time)	DN Menzies
Consultant Endocrinologist (part time)	GM Swyer
Assistants (full time)	DF Hawkins
	BJE Cooke
	FC Hinde
	PEN Suter
Research Anaesthetist	Dr Shila Ransôm
Pathologist	PE Hughesdon
Research Fellows	CN Symth
	GW Theobald
	AH Labrum
Research Assistant (part time)	Mrs Valerie Little

SOURCES

CHAPTER ONE

1. William Nixon's birth certificate, held by Mrs Wendie McWatters.
2. Private correspondence in William Nixon's estate.
3. Bonnici J, Casson M. *The Malta Railway* Valetta: Proudey; 1988.
5. de Bono A. Personal communication (2002). He studied mathematics under Nixon Senior at the University.
6. McWatters W. Personal communication (2001).
7. Elliot P. *The Cross and the Ensign.* St Albans: Grande Publishing; 1982. p.80.
8. Scadding A. Archivist, Epsom College. Personal communication (2002).
9. Bourne, A. Obituary of WCW Nixon, St Mary's Hospital Gazette (1966).

CHAPTER TWO

1. Cope Z. *The History of St Mary's Hospital Medical School.* London: Heineman; 1954.
2. Advertisement in the Medical Directory (1924).
3. Bonney G. Personal communication (2001).
4. Bourne A. *A Doctor's Creed.* London: Victor Gollancz; 1962. p27.
5. Several issues of the St Mary's Hospital Gazette (1923–1927).
6. McWatters W. Personal communication (2002).
7. Bourne A. UCH Gazette (1959).

CHAPTER THREE

1. Personal papers in WCW Nixon's family (1929).
2. Nixon WCW. Calcium therapy and the toxaemias of pregnancy. *Lancet* 1931;**2**:2891–92.
3. Nixon WCW. Influence of age on labour. *Journal of Obstetrics and Gynaecology of the British Empire* 1931;**38**:821–6.
4. Wright H. Fifty years of family planning. *Family Planning* 1972;**17**:40–2.
5. Nixon WCW. Menstruation and its relation to disease. *The Practitioner* 1934;**132**:356–65.
6. McWatters W. Personal communication (2002).

CHAPTER FOUR

1. Mao PWC. *The First Fifty Years of Tsan Yuk Hospital.* Published privately in Hong Kong (1974).

2.   Nixon WCW. Inaugural lecture at University College Hospital (1945).
3.   Nixon WCW. Post-partum haemorrhage. *Chinese Medical Journal* 1936;**50**:1829–34.
4.   Nixon WCW. Lithopaedium. *Journal of Obstetrics and Gynaecology of the British Empire* 1936;**43**:1183–5.
5.   Nixon WCW. Oedema in pregnancy. *Chinese Medical Journal* 1937;**52**:317–28.
6.   Nixon WCW. Oedema in pregnancy. *Journal of Obstetrics and Gynaecology of the British Empire* 1937;**44**:48–59.
7.   Nixon WCW. Aids in the diagnosis and treatment of ectopic gestation. *British Medical Journal* 1937;**2**:579–81.
8.   Nixon WCW. Diagnosis and treatment of disproportion. *The Practitioner* 1939;**142**:163–70.
9.   Caldwell W, Moloy H. Radiological examination of the woman's pelvis in pregnancy, labour and puerperium. *Proceedings of the Royal Society of Medicine* 1938;**32**:5.
10. Nixon WCW. Endometriosis of the bladder. *The Lancet* 1940;**1**:405–6.
11. McCance RA, Nixon WCW. Diet of the expectant mother. *Public Health* 1938;**51**:364–6.

CHAPTER FIVE

1.   Nixon WCW, Wright MD, Ficke EL. Vitamin B1 in urine and placenta in toxaemia of pregnancy. *British Medical Journal* 1942;**1**:605–7.
2.   Nixon WCW. Diet in pregnancy. *Journal of Obstetrics and Gynaecology of the British Empire* 1941;**48**:614–35.
3.   Nixon WCW. Practical application of knowledge of nutrition to pregnancy. *British Medical Bulletin* 1944;**2**:100–1.
4.   McWatters W. Personal communication (2002).
5.   Minutes of the Soho Hospital for Women, Board of Governors (July 1940).
6.   Malta War Museum exhibit on World War Two.
7.   Nixon WCW. Inaugural lecture, University College Hospital (1946).
8.   Nixon WCW. A Turkish interlude. *UCH Magazine* 1953;**38**:11–17.
9.   Hinsley FH. *British Intelligence in the Second World War. The Official History in 6 volumes.* London: HMSO; 1979.
10. McWatters W. Interview with Professor Kazancigil in Istanbul (2003).
11 . Beard R. *A Mary's Man of Exceptional vision.* St Mary's Gazette 1998;**104**:38–40.
12. Hawkins D. Personal communication (2001).
13. Copy of letter of WCW Nixon to his uncle, in Nixon's private correspondence (1945).

14. Nixon WCW Egeli E, Laqueur W, Yahye O. Icterus in pregnancy: a clinico-pathological study including liver biopsy. *Journal of Obstetrics and Gynaecology of the British Empire* 1947;**54**:642–52.

CHAPTER SIX

1. Law B. Personal communication (2003).
2. Read GD. *Revelations of Childbirth*. London: Heineman; 1950.
3. Hawkins D. Personal communication (2001).
4. Royal College of Obstetrics and Gynaecology. Council and Committee Minutes (1953–59).
6. Bourne A. UCH Gazette (1959).
7. Theobald G, Lundberg R. The electrical induction of labour with a transistor pulse generator. *Journal of Obstetrics and Gynaecology of the British Empire* 1956;**69**:434–42.
8. Menzies DN. Personal communication (2003).

CHAPTER SEVEN

1. Swyer G, Daley D. Progesterone implantation in habitual abortion. *British Medical Journal* 1953;**1**:1073–7.
2. Barns HHF, Morgans ME. Pre-diabetic pregnancy. *Journal of Obstetrics and Gynaecology of the British Empire* 1948;**55**:449–54.
3. Swyer G. Hormones and human fertility. *British Medical Bulletin* 1955;**11**:161.
4. Swyer G. Observations on the postcoital test. *Studies on Fertility* 1955;**7**:79.
5. Swyer GI, Lee AE, Masterton JP. Oestrogen excretion in patients with breast cancer. *British Medical Journal* 1961;(**5226**):617–19.
6. Swyer G. Progress in oral contraception. *Bulletin of the Post-Graduate Committee in Medicine, University of Sydney* 1963;**18**:350–63.
7. Smyth N. Personal communication to the author in the Physiology Laboratory at UCL (1948).
8. Smyth N. Experimental electrocardiography of the foetus. *The Lancet* 1953;**1**:1124–6.
9. Smyth N. The guard ring tocograph. *Journal of Obstetrics and Gynaecology of the British Empire* 1957;**64**:59–66.
10. Smyth CN, Wolff HS. Application of endoradiosonde or "wireless pill" to recording of uterine contractions and foetal heart sounds. *The Lancet* 1960;**2**:412–13.
11. Martin J. Personal communication (2002).
12. Smyth N. Effect of valyl oxcytocin on the human subject. *British Medical Journal* 1958;**1**:856–9.

13. Hawkins D. Personal communication (2002).

14. Nixon WCW, Hawkins D. Blood electrolytes in prolonged labour. *Journal of Obstetrics and Gynaecology of the British Empire* 1957;**64**:641–8.

15. Payling-Wright H, Osborn S, Hayden M. Venous velocity in bedridden patients. *The Lancet* 1952;**2**:699–702.

16. Payling-Wright H. Anti-coagulant therapy. *British Medical Journal* 1953;**1**:987–9.

17. Payling-Wright H, Morris N, Osbourn S. Effective circulation in the uterine wall in late pregnancy. *The Lancet* 1953;**1**:323.

18. Payling-Wright H. The effect of diet upon the response to oral anticoagulants. *Journal of Clinical Pathology* 1955;**8**:65.

19. Morris N, Osbourn S, Payling-Wright H, Hart A. The effective uterine bloodflow during exercise in normal and pre-eclamptic pregnancies. *The Lancet* 1956;**2**:481–4.

20. Martin J, Dumoulin J. The use of intravenous Ergometrine to prevent post-partum haemorrhage. *British Medical Journal* 1953;**1**:643–6.

21. Spencer P. Controlled cord traction and management of the third stage of labour. *British Medical Journal* 1962;**1**:1728–32.

22. Bonham D. A preliminary study of the pregnant cervix: antepartum and postpartum. *Proceedings of the Royal Society of Medicine* 1961;**54**:717–20.

23. Bonham DG, Grossman ME, Sidaway ME. Ovarian visualization by gynae-cography. *Proceedings of the Royal Society of Medicine* 1963;**47**:385–60.

24. Bonham D, Gibbs D. A new test for gynaecological cancer and phosphogluconate dehydrogenase activity in vaginal fluid. *British Medical Journal* 1962;**2**:823–4.

25. Skrabanek P. Smoking and statistical overkill. *The Lancet* 1992;**340**:1208–9.

26. Dumoulin J. Personal communication (2002).

27. Nixon WCW. Psychosomatic preparation for childbirth. *Proceedings of the Royal Society of Medicine* 1954;**47**:385–7.

28. Records of Obstetrical Research Committee, University College Hospital (1949).

29. Nixon WCW, Whittet TD. Metric system in medicine and pharmacy. *British Medical Journal* 1953;**1**:327–8.

30. Peel JH. Personal communication, (2002).

31. Fairweather D. Personal communication (2003).

32. Law R. Personal communication (2003).

33. This quotation and the material in this section about the Perinatal Mortality Survey came, with permission, from Dr Susan Williams, Historian to the National Birthday Trust, whose book, *Women and Childbirth in the Twentieth Century*, Sultan Publicity Ltd (1997), is such an excellent account of that Trust's life and death.

34. Philipp E. Personal communication (2002).
35. Bonham D. Personal communication (2003).
36. Butler N, Bonham D. *Perinatal Mortality: The First Report.* Edinburgh: E & S Livingstone; 1963.
37. *The Times* (26 October 1962).
38. *Daily Telegraph* (26 October 1962).
39. *Daily Mirror* 26 October 1962).
40. Butler N, Alberman E. *Periatal Problems: The Second Report.* Edingburgh: E & S Livingstone; 1963.
41. Chamberlain R, Chamberlain G. *British Births 1970.* London: William Heinemann; 1975.
42. Menzies D. Personal communication (2002).

CHAPTER EIGHT
1. *The Medical Directory.* Edinburgh: Churchill Livingstone; 2002.
2. Nordin C, Personal communication (2002).
3. Boyd R. Personal communication (2003).
4. Reports of the Obstetric Department (1955).
5. Blair J. Personal communication (2002).
6. Hawkins D. Personal communication (2002).

CHAPTER NINE
1. Macgregor W. Obituary Notice, WCW Nixon. *British Medical Journal* 1966;**i**:487.
2. Law R. Personal communication.
3. Hawkins D. Personal communication (2002).
4. McWatters W. Personal communication (2002).
5. Williams L. Obituary WCW Nixon. *The Lancet* 1966;**i**:439.
6. Mc Watters W. Personal communication (2002).
7. Documents in the Public Records Office.
8. Flew J. Obituary WCW Nixon. *Journal of Obstetrics and Gynaecology of the British Empire* 1966;**73**:497.
9. Morris N. Obituary WCW Nixon. *British Medical Journal* 1966;**i**:456.
10. Bourne A. Obituary WCW Nixon. *The Lancet* 1966;**i**:439.
11. Phillips E. Personal communication (2002).
12. *The Times* Law Reports 15 April to 5 May 1964.

CHAPTER TEN
1. Menzies D. Personal communication (2002).
2. Hawkins D. Personal communication (2002).

3. Brant H. Personal communication. (2003)
4. Baderman H. Personal communication. (2002).
5. Flew T. Obituary notice WCW Nixon. *The Times* 15 February 1966.
6. Memorial service notice. *Daily Telegraph* 9 April 1966.

INDEX

Stevens, Thomas 18
stilboestrol 53
Suter, PN 69
Swyer, Gerald 53, 71–5
Syntocin® *see* oxytocin

thalidomide 123–5
Theobald, Geoffrey 66–7
Thompson, Angus 89
thrombosis, in pregnancy 54, 80
tocography 75, 83
toxaemia of pregnancy *see* pre–eclampsia
Turkey 39, 40–1, 42–9
Turkish Obstetrical Association 45–6
Turner, Bradwell 3
Tylden, Elizabeth 68

ultrasonography 76–7
University College Hospital (UCH),
Obstetric Unit
    Nixon at 49, 54–5, 58, 61, 62–3, 70–1,
                83, 96, 101, 125, 127
    research at 70–85
    staff 50–61, 63, 64–9, 125–6, 127,
                137–44
Uris, Leon 120–2
Utidjian, Rosemary 126

vaginal examinations 19, 35, 98–9
vesicovaginal fistula 40

Wanklin, Rita 63
Waters, E 82
WellBeing 87
White, Clifford 57
Whittet, Thomas 84
Willcox, Sir William 15
Williams, Cecil 84
Williams, Cicely 61
Wilson, Charles (Lord Moran) 7, 15
women, in medicine 9, 59
Woolf, Anthony 67, 126
World Health Organization (WHO) 62, 65
World War I 7
World War II 38, 40, 41–2
Wright, Almroth 11
Wright, Helena 23–5

X–rays 17, 36, 67

Ysebrand, Vroukje *see* Nixon, Vroukje
Yucel, Dr 72–3